PHARMACOLOGY

A Comprehensive Reference Guide for Medical, Nursing, and Paramedic Students

Review

M. Mastenbjörk M.D.
S. Meloni M.D.

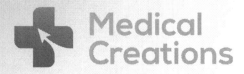

CONTENTS

UNIT VI : THE CARDIOVASCULAR SYSTEM

UNIT VII : HEMATOPOIETIC SYSTEM

UNIT VIII : RESPIRATORY SYSTEM

UNIT IX : GASTROINTESTINAL SYSTEM

UNIT X : GENITOURINARY SYSTEM

UNIT XI : ANTIMICROBIALS

UNIT XII : IMPORTANT MISCELLANEOUS DRUGS

APPENDIX

YOU MIGHT ALSO NEED

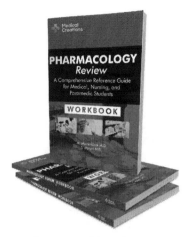

Pharmacology Review:
A Comprehensive Reference
Guide for Medical, Nursing, and
Paramedic Students: Workbook

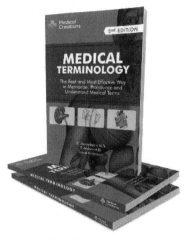

Medical Terminology:
The Best and Most Effective Way
to Memorize, Pronounce and
Understand Medical Terms
(2nd Edition)

Scan the QR Code

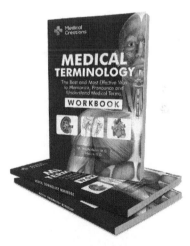

Medical Terminology:
The Best and Most Effective
Way to Memorize, Pronounce
and Understand Medical Terms:
Workbook

FREE GIFT

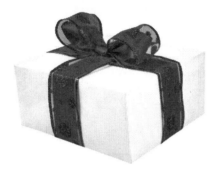

GET ONE OF THESE EBOOKS FOR FREE:

Medical Reference Pamphlet
ACLS ebook
Pulmonology ebook
Neurology ebook
Mini Medical Dictionary
Medical Terminology Digital Pamphlet
ECG - Digital Reference Pamphlet
Pharmacology Digital Pamphlet

Scan the following QR Code:

You will be redirected to our website.
Follow the instructions to claim your free gift.

Introduction

Drug therapy remains the mainstay of treatment in medicine. While physicians prescribe drugs on a daily basis, other healthcare workers also need to familiarize themselves with pharmacology to ensure that the correct dosage regimen is being received by patients, to communicate efficiently with other healthcare workers, and to recognize and deal with adverse effects of pharmacological therapy.

For easy understanding of this complex subject, the book has been divided into multiple units based on each body system. The key therapeutic drug classes for each major system have been outlined in separate chapters. Bullet points and tables make the content easy to understand.

Pharmacology is a constantly evolving field, and new drugs are being developed every day. The main aim of this book is to familiarize the reader with the different categories of drugs. The most commonly prescribed drugs are described here, but the book is by no means exhaustive and does not cover all the drugs available today. For detailed descriptions of the latest drugs on the market, and less commonly prescribed drugs, the reader is referred to one of the more exhaustive textbooks of pharmacology that have been referenced in the text.

UNIT I : THE BASICS

CHAPTER 1

Routes of Drug Administration

For a drug to begin its pharmacological activity, it must first be introduced into the body. This can be done through a variety of routes. Depending on their properties, some drugs can have more than one route of administration.

The ideal route of administration depends on two factors:

- **Properties of the drug** : Whether it is predominantly lipid based or water based, degree of ionization, size of the drug particle, etc.
- **Desired effects of the drug** : Whether the desired effect must be local or systemic, whether immediate or delayed onset of action is desired, etc.

Broadly, there are two main routes of drug administration:

- **Local/Topical** : The drug is intended to act on the site of the body at which it is administered.
- **Systemic** : The drug acts on a site that is away from the area of administration. In the systemic route, the drug needs to be absorbed into the bloodstream, and then be transported to the area where it is intended to act.

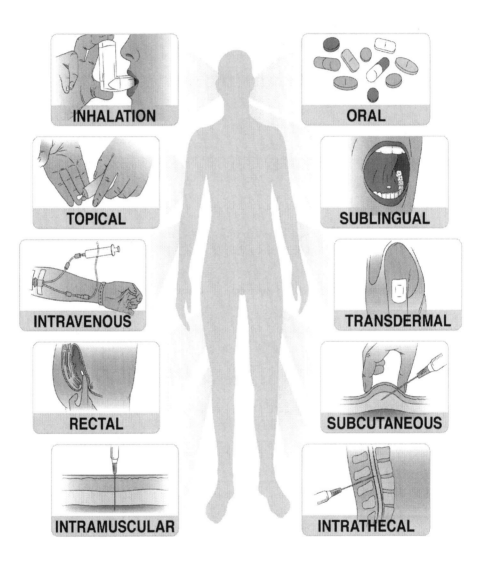

Figure 1 Various routes of drug administration; the ideal route of administration for a particular drug depends on the properties of the drug and the desired effects of the drug.

4

LOCAL ROUTES OF ADMINISTRATION

- **Inhalation** : Inhalation may be oral or nasal. Either way, the drug is delivered directly to the respiratory epithelium. The nasal route is preferred when the action is specifically desired for the nasal epithelium. This route eliminates the risk of systemic side effects. This is useful for patients with respiratory disorders.

- **Intrathecal injection** : The drug is delivered directly into CNS through the cerebrospinal fluid. This is useful for drugs that cannot penetrate the blood-brain barrier. This allows rapid onset of action to take place.

- **Topical** :The drug is directly applied to the surface of the skin. This is used specifically for diseases of the skin and surface mucosa.

SYSTEMIC ROUTES OF ADMINISTRATION

Enteral route:

Enteral refers to administration of the drug through the mouth and gastrointestinal system. This may be oral, sublingual, or rectal.

- **Oral route** : In the oral route, the drug is swallowed, and needs to be absorbed through the gastrointestinal tract. This is the most common route of drug administration.

- **Sublingual and buccal route** : In this route, the drug is placed under the tongue, or in the fold of the cheek. Since these areas have rich vascular supply, the drug is quickly absorbed by the capillaries and sent into systemic circulation.

- **Rectal route** : In this route, the drug is administered through the anal aperture. From here, the drug is absorbed into the external and internal hemorrhoidal veins. The portion of the drug that is absorbed from the external hemorrhoidal veins bypasses the first-pass metabolism.

Parenteral route

In parenteral administration, drugs are directly introduced into systemic circulation. This route is generally suitable for drugs that cannot survive digestive enzymes or first-pass metabolism. The parenteral route requires sterile equipment, in the form of syringes or cannulas, for drug administration.

- **Subcutaneous :** The drug is injected into the loose subcutaneous tissue. This region is not as vascular as other tissues such as the muscle, so absorption into circulation may not be quick. First-pass metabolism is avoided through this route.

- **Intravenous** : The drug is delivered directly into the blood through a vein. Usually, veins of the forearm are cannulated and the drug is delivered. The drug may be given undiluted, which is referred to as a bolus. This delivers

5

the complete drug into the systemic circulation immediately. Alternatively, the drug may be diluted in a carrier such as normal saline, and delivered as an infusion. This allows the drug to be delivered at precise plasma concentrations. The duration of drug action also increases.

- **Intramuscular** : The drug is injected into the muscle. Usually, muscles of the upper arm and shoulder (such as the deltoid) or the pelvic region (such as the gluteus maximus) are selected for intramuscular drug delivery. It is possible to change the rate of absorption of the drug by modifying its carrier solution. Drugs in aqueous solutions are absorbed rapidly, while those in non-aqueous suspensions (called depot preparations) are absorbed slowly. Anticoagulants, such as heparin, cannot be given intramuscularly because they can cause hematomas in the muscle. First-pass metabolism is avoided through this route.

Other systemic routes

- **Transdermal :** The drug is applied to the skin surface. However, from here it gets absorbed through the local vasculature into systemic circulation. Drugs are delivered through the use of skin patches. These patches are stuck onto the skin surface and they remain for a few days to exert their action.

The advantages and disadvantages of the various routes of drug administration are outlined in Table 1.

Table 1. Routes of drug administration

ROUTE OF DRUG ADMINISTRATION	ADVANTAGES	DISADVANTAGES
Inhalation	Rapid absorption and onset of action Lower chances of systemic side effects	Potential for addiction as drug is in close proximity to the brain Requires learning curve to use the inhaler
Intrathecal	Fast and effective route No absorption into systemic circulation, so fewer systemic side effects	Invasive method which requires clinical expertise Chances of inducing or aggravating brain infection if sterility of equipment is compromised
Topical	Non-invasive, painless Convenient Has fewer systemic side effects	Restricted to diseases of the skin and surface mucosa

Sublingual/ Buccal	Most of the advantages of oral route	Effective only for specific drugs that have particular properties, such as high lipid solubility. Otherwise, absorption may be unpredictable.
	The drug does not enter the GIT, so it cannot be affected by digestive enzymes. Avoidance first-pass metabolism by the liver.	One must be careful not to swallow the drug
	Absorption is rapid and the onset of action is fast.	
Oral	Convenient and cost-effective. Does not require medical assistance and sterile equipment such as syringes.	Requires patient cooperation. Oral administration is difficult if the patient is unconscious, or is vomiting.
	Painless	Some drugs may be subjected to degradation by digestive enzymes. This may be avoided by the use of enteric-coated preparations.
	Toxicity can easily be reversed through gastric lavage. This is useful if the drug does not have a specific antidote.	Absorption of the drug from the GIT is often unpredictable. To a certain extent, this can be controlled through the use of extended-release preparations.
		Slow onset of action. Hence, not suitable for emergencies.
Subcutaneous	Bypasses GIT and metabolic pathways	Invasive method
	Can be self-administered with practice	Only small volumes of drug can be administered.
	Effects are slow, sustained and predictable	

Rectal	50% of the drug bypasses first-pass metabolism. The entire drug, however, escapes the action of digestive enzymes. Absorption is rapid, resulting in faster onset of action It can be used in unconscious patients, as well as patients with vomiting.	Requires cooperation in the conscious patient. Administering the drug through this route may be associated with some discomfort. Drug absorption is erratic and unpredictable.
Intravenous	Immediate onset of action is achieved, suitable for emergencies Bypasses GIT and metabolic pathways The quantity of drug delivered can be precisely controlled	Invasive and painful route, requires trained medical personnel Potential for infection by contamination at the injection site Irritant drugs may cause thrombophlebitis Difficult to treat toxicities unless a specific antidote exists
Intramuscular	Bypasses GIT and metabolic pathways Can control rate of absorption	Invasive method, cannot be self-administered Can cause muscle spasm or pain, especially with non-aqueous preparations Not advisable in patients who are taking anticoagulants, as it can cause internal hemorrhage.
Transdermal	Bypasses GIT and metabolic pathways Painless and convenient	Patches can cause skin irritation Only suitable for lipophilic drugs, in small doses.

EXERCISES

1. Which of the following routes must be avoided in patients on anticoagulants?
   a. Subcutaneous
   b. Oral
   c. Intramuscular
   d. Transdermal

2. Which of the following routes does not completely bypass the first-pass metabolism of the liver?
   a. Sublingual
   b. Transdermal
   c. Rectal
   d. Subcutaneous

3. Which of the following routes is most effective in delivering the drug directly into systemic circulation?
   a. Intravenous
   b. Intramuscular
   c. Subcutaneous
   d. Sublingual

4. Which of the following routes is ideal for treating CNS infections with a drug that cannot penetrate the blood brain barrier?
   a. Intravenous
   b. Intrathecal
   c. Sublingual
   d. Inhalational

5. Which of the following routes is meant to work by transferring drugs into systemic circulation?
   a. Inhalational
   b. Intrathecal
   c. Topical
   d. Transdermal

6. Which of the following routes is ideal for patients with respiratory infections?
   a. Intramuscular
   b. Inhalational
   c. Intrathecal
   d. Intravenous

7. In the intramuscular route, which muscle is preferred for injection?
   a. Gluteus minimus
   b. Gluteus intermedius
   c. Gluteus maximus
   d. Piriformis

8. Which of the following routes of administration does not require the use of sterile equipment?
   a. Subcutaneous
   b. Sublingual
   c. Intravenous
   d. Intramuscular

9. Which of the following routes of administration is safest for drugs where no known antidote exists?
   a. Oral
   b. Sublingual
   c. Rectal
   d. Intramuscular

10. In which of the following routes is the drug absorbed through hemorrhoidal veins?
    a. Sublingual
    b. Rectal
    c. Intravenous
    d. Intramuscular

CHAPTER 2

Pharmacokinetics and Pharmacodynamics

The science of pharmacology basically deals with the interaction of the drug with the body. This has two main divisions: Pharmacokinetics, which describes what the body does to the drug; and Pharmacodynamics, which describes what the drug does to the body.

PHARMACOKINETICS

To put it simply, pharmacokinetics describes the journey of the drug through the body. Once the drug enters the body, it goes through the following phases until it is eliminated:

- **Absorption** : The drug enters the bloodstream from the tissue in which it was administered. This phase is only applicable for drugs that are administered through the systemic route.
- **Distribution** : The drug leaves the bloodstream and enters the body tissues. It is in this phase that most drugs exert their clinical effects. This includes both intended biological effects and adverse effects.
- **Metabolism** : The body acts on the drug to metabolize it. Metabolism may either degrade the drug, making it inactive, or may convert an inactive drug form into its active form. In the latter case, clinical effects take place after metabolism.
- **Elimination** : This is the phase where the drug, either in its original form, or metabolized form, leaves the body.

Absorption

Once the drug enters into the body, it must move from the tissue in which it was administered, into the bloodstream. This process is referred to as absorption. The amount of drug that is absorbed, and the rate of absorption generally depend on several factors:

- The environment (for instance, pH) from which absorption must take place
- Route of administration
- Properties of the drug

The extent to which a drug is absorbed is referred to as 'bioavailability'. Only the bioavailable drug is available for clinical effect; the rest is excreted without absorption. Drugs administered through intravenous routes have 100% bioavailability. Other parenteral routes may have slightly less bioavailability because of some amount of local binding. However, the oral route often has decreased bioavailability. The following section, therefore, focuses on absorption of drugs from the GIT.

Methods of drug absorption from the GIT:

When ingested orally, the drugs must pass from within the GIT, through the walls of the epithelium, into systemic circulation. This is achieved by one of the following methods:

- **Passive diffusion** : The drug moves naturally from an area of high concentration to the area of low concentration. Lipid soluble drugs pass easily through the phospholipid bilayer of the cell membrane, while water soluble drugs use aqueous channels to penetrate through the cell membrane.
- **Facilitated diffusion** : Some drugs bind to specialized proteins called transmembrane carrier proteins. These proteins change their configuration and allow drugs to pass through them from areas of higher to lower concentration.
- **Active transport** : The drug moves against a concentration gradient, from areas of low to high concentration. This requires energy, which is obtained by hydrolysis of adenosine triphosphate (ATP). Drugs that are structurally similar to naturally occurring metabolites in the body may require active transport.
- **Endocytosis** : The drug is engulfed into a portion of the cell membrane, which pinches off from the rest of the membrane to form a vesicle. This vesicle is transported inside the cell, and the drug is released. This process occurs when the drug has a large molecular size.

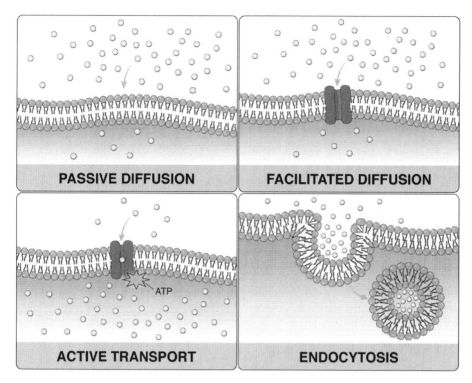

Figure 2 Drugs that are ingested orally end up in systemic circulation by passive diffusion, facilitated diffusion, active transport, or endocytosis.

Factors that affect absorption of the drug from the GIT:

- **pH of the external environment and the pKa of the drug** : Together, these two factors determine the ratio of the unionized to the ionized form of the drug. A drug that has a low pKa (or is acidic) tends to have a higher amount of unionized form when the surrounding pH is low. A drug that has a high pKa (or is basic) tends to have a higher proportion of unionized form when the surrounding pH is high. Only the unionized form is capable of diffusing through the intestinal membranes.

- **Blood flow at the site of absorption** : More vascularized regions of the GIT tend to absorb drugs faster. The intestines are more vascular than the stomach, so drugs are absorbed faster here.

- **Surface area available for absorption** : Absorption is more efficient over a larger surface area. The epithelium lining the small intestine has microvilli, which greatly increases the surface area available. This makes the absorption here more efficient than in the stomach.

Factors affecting bioavailability from the oral route of administration:

- **First-pass metabolism** : After absorption from the GIT, before the drug can enter systemic circulation, it first passes through portal circulation. During this passage, the drug might become metabolized by the liver. This is referred to as first-pass metabolism, and this limits the bioavailability of several drugs.

- **Resistance to digestive enzymes** : Some drugs may not survive degradation by digestive enzymes, which limits their availability.

- **Solubility of the drug** : A drug that is highly lipid soluble may find it difficult to gain access to the cell surface. At the same time, a highly hydrophilic drug cannot permeate the phospholipid bilayer. Ideally, the drug should be lipophilic, with some amount of hydrophilic nature.

DISTRIBUTION

During distribution, the drug leaves the bloodstream and enters the extracellular fluid and tissues. This is a reversible process, and the drug can re-enter the bloodstream, only to be re-distributed to other tissues. Drugs administered through the intravenous route skip the absorption phase and are directly distributed to tissues.

Factors affecting distribution:

- **Vascularity of tissues** : Organs with high blood supply (such as the brain, liver, and kidney) receive the drug first. Tissues such as the skeletal muscle come next, while the adipose tissue, skin, and other organs have lower blood flow and therefore receive the drug more slowly.

- **Capillary permeability** : Capillary permeability refers to the ability of the blood vessel wall to allow molecules to pass through them. If the endothelial cells in the vessel wall have numerous slit junctions between them, permeability is high, and the drug can easily pass out of circulation into the tissues. The liver and spleen, for instance, have high capillary permeability. If there are no slit junctions, capillary permeability is low. The brain has tight endothelial cell-to-cell contact, referred to as the blood-brain barrier. Therefore, some drugs cannot penetrate easily into the brain tissue.

- **Binding of the drug to plasma protein** : The main plasma protein involved in drug-binding is albumin. If the drug is in the bound form, the entire drug may not get distributed into the tissue. Some drugs remain bound to albumin, and serve as a reservoir. This is released when the free drug is redistributed or eliminated.

- **Binding of the drug to tissue protein** : The drug may bind to various proteins in the tissue and serve as a reservoir here. This tends to avoid redistribution, and may prolong the action of the drug.

14

- **Lipid solubility** : Only lipophilic drugs can penetrate the phospholipid bilayer of the cell membrane. Hydrophilic drugs, on the other hand, cannot penetrate cell membranes, and must cross the membrane through slit junctions.

METABOLISM

Metabolism serves two purposes. Firstly, the active drug may be converted into a form that is easier to eliminate from the body. This may or may not result in inactivation of the drug. Secondly, the drug may be inactive to begin with, but metabolism may convert the drug into an active form. Further metabolism may be needed to prepare the drug for elimination. Most drugs undergo metabolism in the liver, but some metabolism can occur in the plasma, GIT, or other organs. Metabolism involves two specific phases:

Phase I reactions

This involves conversion of lipophilic drugs into hydrophilic, or polar molecules, which can easily be excreted by the kidney. This is achieved by three kinds of reactions – reduction, oxidation, and hydrolysis. This is achieved through two methods:

- **Reactions involving the cytochrome P450 system** : The P450 is a superfamily of isozymes that contain heme. This system is present in most cells, but is especially abundant in the liver and GIT. While there are several distinct isozymes, four play an important role in drug metabolism. These include CYP3A4/5, CYP2D6, CYP2C8/9 and CYP1A2.
- **Reactions not involving the P450 system** : These include amine oxidation, alcohol dehydrogenation, esterases, and hydrolysis reactions.

Phase II reactions

If sufficient polarity is not achieved through Phase I metabolism, the drugs enter into Phase II reactions. These are conjugation reactions, where the drug is combined with a naturally occurring substrate, such as acetic acid or glucuronic acid.

ELIMINATION

After metabolism, the drug is eliminated from the body. Elimination usually occurs through the kidneys in the form of urine. Other routes of elimination include the bile and feces, exhaled air, and breast milk.

Renal elimination of drugs

Sufficiently polarized drugs are usually eliminated through the kidney. Like other metabolic products, the drug has to pass through the following phases prior to excretion:

- **Glomerular filtration** : This takes place at the glomerular capillary plexus. Unbound drug molecules can pass from the bloodstream through capillary

15

slit junctions into the glomerular filtrate. The only factor which affects this process is the degree of plasma protein binding of the drug. Bound molecules cannot enter the filtrate.

- **Proximal tubular secretion** : Drugs which were not filtered at the glomerular level enter the plexus surrounding the proximal tubule. Here, some drugs can be secreted into the filtrate by an energy-based active transport system.

- **Distal tubular reabsorption** : Some quantity of the drug may be reabsorbed into the bloodstream at this level. Reabsorption is passive and occurs along a concentration gradient.

Other routes of drug elimination

- **Feces :** Drugs that are secreted into the bile after metabolism, and drugs that are not absorbed via the oral route of administration are eliminated through the feces.

- **Exhaled air** : Drugs delivered through inhalation are also usually eliminated through this route.

- **Body fluids :** Small quantities of drugs may be eliminated through sweat, saliva, and tears. Elimination through breast milk is significant because it may cause unnecessary exposure of the feeding infant to the drug, which may result in undesirable adverse effects.

Measures of drug clearance from the body

To calculate the optimum dosing regimen, and to avoid toxicity, it is important to measure drug clearance from the body. There are two important measures of drug clearance:

Total body clearance : This is the sum of all clearances from the organs that metabolize drugs, and the organs that eliminate drugs. So this is usually hepatic clearance plus renal clearance, but may include clearance from lungs and other organs where applicable.

Drug half-life : Drug half-life, or t1/2, is the unit of time in which the plasma drug concentration decreases by 50%. Factors that affect t1/2 include diminished renal or hepatic blood flow, diminished renal function, and hepatic insufficiency. These can increase the t1/2, and prolong drug action. It takes five cycles of t1/2 for the drug to be completely eliminated from the body.

PHARMACODYNAMICS

Pharmacodynamics refers to the clinical effect that the drug has on the body, or, to put it simply, how the drug works. There are basically three methods by which drugs can exert their effects on the body:

- **Through physical properties** : Some drugs provide a bulking function (e.g., Laxatives like Psyllium husk), or lubricating or coating function (e.g., Dimethicone). These physical properties produce clinical effects.

- **Through chemical properties** : Certain drugs work by chemical reactions. For instance, some drugs work by neutralization of pH (e.g., Antacids), or by their chelating properties (e.g., EDTA).

- **Through receptor binding** : This is the most common method through which drugs exert their effects. In this method, drugs interact with specific receptor proteins present on the surface of the cell. Once the drug binds with the receptor, it is capable of bringing about biochemical changes, or molecular activity that causes the clinical effects of the drug.

Types of receptors

All receptors are proteins that extend through the thickness of the cell membrane. There are essentially four classes of receptors with which drugs interact. These are as follows:

- **Transmembrane ligand-gated ion channels** : 'Ligand-gated' means that the functioning of the ion channel (opening or closing) depends on the binding of specific molecules, called ligands. The ligand binding site is located on the outside. When the ligand (or drug) binds to the channel, the gate opens, allowing influx or efflux of ions. Ionic flow across the membrane can mediate multiple functions, including nerve impulse transmission and muscle contraction.

- **Transmembrane G-protein-coupled receptors** : Like ion channels, the ligand binding site is located on the external side. When the ligand binds to the receptor, the inner part of the receptor interacts with G-proteins, causing them to dissociate. The G-protein subunits in turn activate other intracellular enzymes or proteins, to produce molecular changes.

- **Enzyme-linked receptors** : When the drug binds to this class of receptors, the receptors undergo conformational changes, which increases the activity of intracellular enzymes. This in turn activates other intracellular signals, and a cascade of activity will result.

- **Intracellular receptors** : This is different from other receptors because the drug binding site is located within the cell. So, for the drug to bind to the receptor, it must diffuse across the cell membrane (which requires sufficient lipid solubility). The drug-receptor complex usually translocates to the nucleus, where it binds to transcription factors. This may modify transcription of RNA or DNA and protein translation.

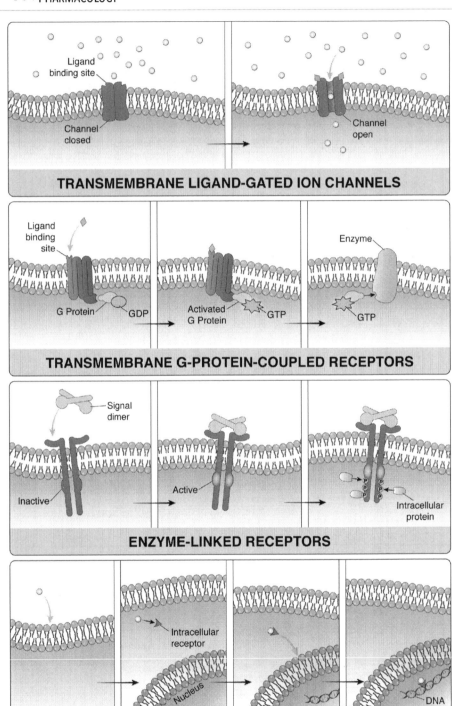

TRANSMEMBRANE LIGAND-GATED ION CHANNELS

TRANSMEMBRANE G-PROTEIN-COUPLED RECEPTORS

ENZYME-LINKED RECEPTORS

INTRACELLULAR RECEPTORS

Figure 3 Drugs may exert their effects by binding to receptors, proteins that extend through the cell membrane. The four types of drug receptors are transmembrane ligand-gated ion channels, transmembrane G-protein-coupled receptors, enzyme-linked receptors, and intracellular receptors.

Effect of drug on the receptors

Not all drugs interact with the receptors in the same way. The actions of the drug may mimic that of substances within the body (endogenous ligands), or may oppose these actions. Depending on the effects that they produce as compared to endogenous ligands, the drugs may be categorized as follows:

- **Full agonists** : If the drug produces the same response as the endogenous ligand, and achieves maximum biological response, it is termed a full agonist.

- **Partial agonists** : The drug may produce the same response as an endogenous ligand, but cannot achieve maximum biological response.

- **Inverse agonists** : Some receptors may get activated spontaneously in the absence of ligand binding. Inverse agonists act on such receptors to deactivate them and bring them to their resting state.

- **Antagonists :** The drug has a high affinity for the receptor site and binds to it. However, it fails to have any effect on the receptor. In the absence of an agonist (either endogenous, or drug), the antagonist has no effect. However, if the agonist is also present, the antagonist can reduce its clinical activity in one of the following ways:

  o Competition: The agonist and antagonist compete for the same binding site on the receptor.
  o Irreversible binding : The antagonist binds irreversibly with the binding site of the receptor, which reduces the receptors available to the agonist for binding.
  o Allosteric binding : The antagonist binds to a different site than the agonist, but prevents receptor activation.
  o Functional antagonism : The antagonist binds to a completely different receptor, but initiates actions that are opposite to the effects of the agonist.

EXERCISES
---

1. In which of the following forms of absorption does the drug move against a concentration gradient?
   a. Facilitated diffusion
   b. Active transport
   c. Passive diffusion
   d. Endocytosis

2. Which of the following is a hindrance to distribution of the drug within the tissues?
   a. Increased tissue protein binding capacity
   b. Increased lipid solubility
   c. Increased plasma protein binding capacity
   d. Increased vascularity of the tissues

3. Which of the following is a Phase II reaction of drug metabolism?
   a. Oxidation
   b. Alcohol dehydrogenation
   c. Conjugation
   d. Hydrolysis

4. How many half-lives of the drug must complete for the drug to be completely eliminated from the body?
   a. Two
   b. Three
   c. Four
   d. Five

5. Which of the following types of drugs has no effect on the receptor when used alone?
   a. Full agonist
   b. Partial agonist
   c. Inverse agonist
   d. Antagonist

6. Which of the following drugs will be absorbed faster from the stomach (low PH)?
   a. Low pKa
   b. High pKa
   c. Neutral pKa
   d. pKa does not matter

7. Which of the following drugs deactivates the receptor upon binding?
   a. Full agonist
   b. Partial agonist
   c. Inverse agonist
   d. Antagonist

8. How does EDTA produce clinical effects?
   a. Through physical properties
   b. Through chemical properties
   c. Through receptors
   d. A combination of the above

9. Which class of receptors induces changes in DNA?
   a. Ligand-gated
   b. G-protein-coupled
   c. Enzyme-linked
   d. Intracellular

10. What protein does the cytochrome P450 system have?
   a. Albumin
   b. Heme
   c. Ferritin
   d. Ceruloplasmin

UNIT II : CENTRAL NERVOUS SYSTEM

CHAPTER 1

General Anesthetics

The term anesthesia refers to loss of sensation. 'General' anesthesia is the term used when loss of sensation is accompanied by loss of consciousness. General anesthesia is applied during interventional medical and surgical procedures. It not only avoids an uncomfortable experience for the patient, it also makes the process easier for the surgeon. With general anesthesia, the following effects are obtained:

- Suppressed or complete loss of consciousness
- Amnesia and reduction in anxiety levels
- Suppression of pain (analgesia) and other sensations
- Suppression of reflexes
- Skeletal muscle relaxation

No single drug is capable of producing all the above effects. Therefore, a group of drugs is combined before and during the anesthetic procedure, in order to achieve all the desired effects.

PREANESTHETIC MEDICATION

To smoothen the process of anesthesia and decrease its side effects, certain drugs are given prior to the procedure. A brief description of the drugs used in pre-anesthetic medication follows. A detailed description of each drug will be described in the relevant chapters.

- **Anticholinergic drugs** : Glycopyrrolate is the most commonly used drug. Its uses are mainly to prevent bradycardia and hypotension that can occur due to vagal stimulation. It also helps prevent laryngospasm that can occur due to respiratory secretions.

- **H2 blockers and proton pump inhibitors** : H2 blockers such as ranitidine, or proton pump inhibitors such as omeprazole may be given the night before, or on the morning of the procedure. They raise the pH of gastric secretions, and prevent regurgitation. They can also prevent stress ulcers.

- **Antiemetics** : These help decrease the incidence of postoperative nausea and vomiting, which is a side effect of several anesthetic agents. Commonly used antiemetic agents include ondansetron, metoclopramide, and domperidone.

- **Sedative/hypnotic drugs, and opioids** : These drugs allay anxiety, and help smoothen induction of anesthesia. Opioids also provide analgesia.

STAGES OF GENERAL ANESTHESIA

- **Induction** : This is the time taken from the administration of the anesthetic agent, to the time the anesthetic agent takes effect. Induction is generally done using intravenous drugs. These drugs act within 30 to 40 seconds, to produce loss of consciousness.

- **Maintenance** : Once anesthesia has been achieved, it must be maintained at the desired depth. This is done using inhalational drugs. The depth of anesthesia is characterized by four different stages:

  o **Stage 1- Analgesia** : The patient loses pain sensation, and may feel drowsy. Respiration and reflexes are intact.

  o **Stage 2- Excitement and delirium** : Blood pressure and respiratory rate increase due to excitement. This stage may be suppressed with rapid acting induction agents.

  o **Stage 3- Surgical anesthesia** : Respiration becomes regular, there is gradual loss of muscle tone and skeletal muscle relaxation occurs. As this stage progresses, first the corneal and laryngeal reflexes, and then the light reflexes are lost. The stage ends with loss of spontaneous breathing. This is the stage where surgery is carried out, and the anesthetist must monitor the patient continuously to prevent progression to stage 4.

  o **Stage 4- Medullary paralysis** : The respiratory and vasomotor centers of the medulla are depressed. The patient will require ventilator and circulatory support to survive.

- **Recovery** : This is essentially the reverse of induction. Inhalational gases are withdrawn and the patient is allowed to return to consciousness. Reversal agents may be required for removing neuromuscular blockage caused by skeletal muscle relaxants.

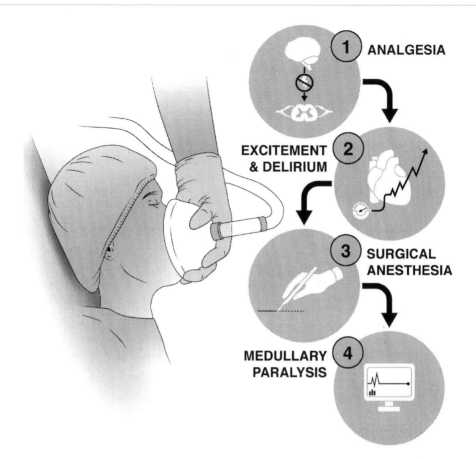

Figure 4 Anesthesia must be maintained at the desired depth once achieved. The depth of anesthesia is characterized by four stages: analgesia, excitement and delirium, surgical anesthesia, and medullary paralysis.

DRUGS USED TO OBTAIN GENERAL ANESTHESIA

In general, there are two classes of drugs that are used for general anesthesia. Intravenous drugs are primarily used for the induction process, while inhalational drugs are used for maintenance of anesthesia.

INHALATIONAL AGENTS

General features of most inhaled anesthetics:

- **State** : Inhalational agents are always gaseous. They are usually non-flammable and non-explosive.

- **Minimum alveolar concentration (MAC)** : This is defined as the concentration of anesthetic needed to eliminate responsive movement to incision in at least

50% of the patients. MAC is inversely related to potency, and therefore, highly potent anesthetics have low MAC values, and vice versa.

- **Pharmacokinetics :** Most inhaled anesthetics go through the following stages:

  o **Alveolar wash-in :** This is the stage where the normal gases in the lung are pushed out and replaced with the anesthetic. The time required for this is directly proportional to the functional residual capacity of the lung, and is inversely proportional to the ventilator rate.

  o **Uptake of anesthetic by tissues :** The anesthetic is carried by the blood from the lungs to peripheral tissues, where it is taken up. The following factors affect anesthetic uptake:

    - Solubility: Drugs with low solubility move in and out of tissues rapidly. So induction and recovery is faster.
    - Cardiac output: High cardiac output prevents faster saturation of blood with anesthetic, and slows induction.
    - Vascularity: Highly vascular tissues such as the brain, heart, liver, and kidney take up the drug first, followed by skeletal muscles. Poorly perfused tissues such as fat and bone do not receive the anesthetic.

  o **Washout :** This is the reverse of wash-in. When the anesthetic is discontinued, the gas is gradually replaced by normal lung gases and the patient recovers.

- **Mechanism of action :** The mechanism of action of most anesthetics is still unclear. These gases appear to act at a variety of receptors. Most anesthetics work at the GABA (γ-amino butyric acid) receptor, and increase the receptor's sensitivity to GABA, which is an inhibitory neurotransmitter. Other anesthetics (for example, nitrous oxide and ketamine), inhibit the NMDA (N-methyl D-aspartate) receptor's sensitivity to glutamate, which is an excitatory neurotransmitter.

Halothane:

- This is the prototype anesthetic. It provides rapid induction and quick recovery.
- Effect on body systems:

  o Potent bronchodilator. It is non-pungent, and has a pleasant odor.
  o Relaxation of skeletal and uterine muscles; therefore, useful in obstetrics

- Adverse effects:

  o Halothane hepatitis: The metabolites of halothane are toxic hydrocarbons that, in selected adult patients, can cause hepatitis and hepatic necrosis.
  o Cardiac effects : It can cause bradycardia and cardiac arrhythmias. It may cause concentration-dependent hypotension.
  o Malignant hyperthermia : This can occur in a small percentage of patients. There is an uncontrolled increase in skeletal muscle metabolism, resulting

26

in dangerously high body temperatures, and inability to supply oxygen and remove carbon dioxide. The antidote, dantrolene sodium, must be used immediately to reverse this, and the drug must be withdrawn immediately.

Isoflurane:

- Has higher blood solubility, so produces slower onset of action and recovery.
- Does not metabolize, so risk of hepatitis is low.
- Like halothane, it produces concentration-dependent hypotension.
- Stimulates respiratory reflexes like cough and laryngospasm, due to its pungent odor.

Desflurane:

- Has the lowest blood solubility of all anesthetics, so has very rapid induction and recovery. It is very suited for outpatient procedures.
- Minimal tissue toxicity.
- Also stimulates respiratory reflexes, and has low volatility, so it needs to be administered through a special heated vaporizer.

Sevoflurane:

- Solubility is higher than desflurane and nitrous oxide, but still allows quick induction and recovery.
- Non-pungent, does not stimulate respiratory reflexes.
- Undergoes metabolism like halothane, but its metabolites may be nephrotoxic.

Nitrous oxide:

- This has a high MAC and weak potency.
- It is poorly soluble in blood, and can therefore move in and out of tissues rapidly.
- Effects on body systems:
  o Does not depress respiration.
  o Does not cause muscle relaxation.
  o Does not affect the cardiovascular system.
  o Does not increase cerebral blood flow.
  o Least hepatotoxic of all inhaled anesthetics.

These properties make it the safest of all anesthetics, although it is the least potent.

- Adverse effects: Because of its rapid movement, it can retard uptake of oxygen during recovery, leading to diffusion hypoxia. This can be avoided by using large volumes of oxygen.

INTRAVENOUS AGENTS

General features of intravenous anesthetics

- **Pharmacokinetics :** Because they are injected intravenously, these drugs have 100% bioavailability. The drug passes from the injected vein, though the heart, into systemic circulation, and is then delivered to the brain. Diffusibility into the brain depends on degree of plasma protein binding, degree of ionization, and lipid solubility. Unbound, unionized, and lipid soluble drugs penetrate the brain faster. After initially flooding the brain, the drug gets rapidly redistributed to other tissues like skeletal muscles, resulting in rapid recovery from anesthesia.

- **Mechanism of action :** Like inhalational anesthetics, the exact mechanism of action is unknown, but it is probably similar to that of the inhalational agents.

Based on the time of onset of action, there are two classes of intravenous agents – fast-acting agents and slower-acting agents.

FAST-ACTING INTRAVENOUS ANESTHETICS

The fast-acting drugs are generally used for induction of general anesthesia. These drugs can also be used as the sole anesthetic agent for short procedures.

Propofol:

- Induction occurs within 30-40 seconds after administration. Redistribution half–life is within 2 to 4 minutes. These are unaltered in hepatic and renal failure.
- Effects on body systems:
  - o Causes systemic vasodilation, which decreases blood pressure and intracranial pressure.
  - o Occasionally can cause excitation, such as muscle twitching, hiccups, and spontaneous movement.
  - o Can cause sedation alone in lower doses.
  - o Has an antiemetic effect, so associated with lower incidence of postoperative nausea and vomiting.
  - o Does not provide analgesia.

Thiopental:

- This is an ultra-short-acting barbiturate. It produces induction in 15-20 seconds. Redistribution half-life is 3 minutes.
- Effects on body systems:
  - o Decrease in blood pressure and intracranial pressure. Can cause severe hypotension in patients with shock.
  - o Can cause laryngospasm and bronchospasm if the airway is irritated.

28

o It is a poor analgesic.

SLOWER-ACTING INTRAVENOUS ANESTHETICS

Benzodiazepines:

- These are primarily sedative-hypnotic drugs. The properties of these drugs are described in detail in Chapter 2.

- When these drugs are used in larger doses (as compared to their sedative-hypnotic dose), they may be used as anesthetic agents. The more commonly used benzodiazepines for this purpose are as follows:

  o Diazepam: Diazepam produces unconsciousness in 15 to 30 minutes. Redistribution half-life is 15 minutes. The sedative effect, however, lasts for at least six hours.

  o Midazolam: This is preferred to diazepam as an anesthetic as it is faster, and short-acting. It is three times more potent than diazepam.

  o Lorazepam: It is as potent as midazolam, however, is slower-acting and causes slower onset and recovery.

Opioids:

- Certain opioids, including fentanyl, sufentanil, and remifentanil are often used as anesthetic agents. All opioids can lead to hypotension, respiratory depression, muscle rigidity, and postoperative nausea and vomiting. Naloxone can be used as an antagonist of opioid effects. The properties of opioids are described in greater detail in Chapter 3.

- Since they are analgesics, they are preferred for painful procedures, such as angiography and endoscopic procedures. The combination of morphine and nitrous oxide provides good anesthesia for cardiac surgery. However, they do not produce amnesia, and are therefore combined with benzodiazepines for better patient comfort.

- Fentanyl can cause bradycardia and respiratory depression. It increases muscle tone, and must therefore be combined with muscle relaxants to facilitate mechanical ventilation.

Ketamine:

- Ketamine produces a unique state of anesthesia referred to as dissociative anesthesia. In this state, the patient appears to be awake (eyes open, muscles are stiff, and may swallow); but the patient is unconscious, and there is immobility, amnesia, and profound analgesia.

- The drug is highly lipophilic and rapidly enters the cerebral cortex and subcortical areas. It quickly redistributes and is metabolized in the liver. Elimination half-life is two to four hours.

- There is cardiac stimulation, with increased blood pressure and cardiac output. It is contraindicated in hypertensive patients. On the other hand, it produces bronchodilation, and is beneficial for use in asthmatics. However, increased cerebral blood flow and postoperative hallucinations have restricted its use.

Etomidate:

- This is a short-acting hypnotic agent that provides rapid induction. It has poor analgesic activity.
- It does not have any effect on the cardiovascular system, and is therefore suitable in patients with cardiovascular disease.
- Etomidate suppresses plasma cortisol and aldosterone levels, and therefore should not be infused for extended periods of time.

Dexmedetomidine:

- This drug functions by activating the central $\alpha2$ adrenergic receptors. It produces both sedation and analgesia.
- This drug does not cause respiratory depression, and blunts cardiovascular response to stress.
- It has relatively minor side effects, including dry mouth, hypotension, and bradycardia.

EXERCISES

1. Which of the following pre-anesthetic medications helps to prevent laryngospasm?
    a. Ranitidine
    b. Glycopyrrolate
    c. Pantoprazole
    d. Metoclopramide

2. In which of the following stages of general anesthesia must surgical procedures be carried out?
    a. Stage 1
    b. Stage 2
    c. Stage 3
    d. Stage 4

3. Which of the following inhalational anesthetics is associated with malignant hyperthermia?
    a. Halothane
    b. Isoflurane
    c. Desflurane
    d. Sevoflurane

4. Which of the following intravenous anesthetic agents produces the phenomenon called dissociative anesthesia?
    a. Fentanyl
    b. Thiopental
    c. Midazolam
    d. Ketamine

5. Which of the following anesthetic agents is suitable for patients with cardiovascular disease?
    a. Midazolam
    b. Etomidate
    c. Fentanyl
    d. Propofol

6. Which of the following anesthetic gases is non-pungent and has a pleasant odor?
   a. Halothane
   b. Sevoflurane
   c. Desflurane
   d. Isoflurane

7. Which of the following anesthetics can cause diffusion hypoxia?
   a. Halothane
   b. Nitrous oxide
   c. Midazolam
   d. Sevoflurane

8. Which of the following agents has maximum analgesic effect?
   a. Fentanyl
   b. Diazepam
   c. Thiopental
   d. Propofol

9. Which of the following anesthetics has an anti-emetic effect?
   a. Fentanyl
   b. Diazepam
   c. Thiopental
   d. Propofol

10. Which of the following is the least hepatotoxic?
   a. Halothane
   b. Sevoflurane
   c. Nitrous oxide
   d. Isoflurane

CHAPTER 2

Sedative-Hypnotic Drugs

Sedatives (also known as anti-anxiety or anxiolytic drugs) are agents that depress excitement and calm the patient. Although sedatives can cause some drowsiness, they do not induce sleep or loss of consciousness. Hypnotics are drugs that induce normal, arousable sleep, as opposed to loss of consciousness induced by general anesthetics. Some drugs can function as sedatives at lower doses, and as hypnotics at higher doses.

There are three main classes of sedative and hypnotic agents:

- Benzodiazepines
- Barbiturates
- Other drugs (sometimes referred to as non-benzodiazepine hypnotics)

BENZODIAZEPINES

Benzodiazepines are the most commonly used sedative-hypnotic drugs today.

Mechanism of action:

Benzodiazepines act at the GABA receptor. GABA (γ- amino butyric acid) is an inhibitory neurotransmitter. When GABA binds to its receptor, chloride channels open, allowing influx of chloride into the cell, which causes hyperpolarization of the neuron. This prevents development of an action potential. Benzodiazepines increase the affinity of GABA for its receptor, potentiating this action.

Clinical effects:

- Reduction of anxiety and sedation at lower doses, hypnosis at higher doses.
- **Anterograde amnesia** : Benzodiazepines impair the ability to form new memories.
- Anticonvulsant activity
- Muscle relaxation

33

Pharmacokinetics:

- Route of administration is generally oral.

- All benzodiazepines are lipophilic to some degree, but there is some variation between the different drugs. This affects the rate of absorption, and duration of action of the drug. Based on the duration of action, benzodiazepines may be classified as short-acting, intermediate-acting, or long-acting drugs. (Table 1)

- The t 1/2 does not correlate with the clinical duration of action. This is because even the unmetabolized drug may dissociate from the receptor and redistribute to other tissues of the body.

- Most benzodiazepines are metabolized in the liver by the hepatic microsomal system (CYP3A4 and CYP2C19 enzymes) to glucuronides oxidized metabolites.

- Excretion occurs through the urine.

- Benzodiazepines can cross the placental barrier and depress the fetal CNS. It can also be secreted in breast milk. Therefore, it is not recommended for pregnant and nursing women.

Table 1. Classification of benzodiazepines based on duration of action.

DRUG CATEGORY	DRUG EXAMPLES	T ½ (HOURS)	CLINICAL DOSE
Long-acting (less lipophilic)	Flurazepam	50-100	15mg to 30 mg
	Diazepam	30-60	5mg to 10 mg
Intermediate-acting	Alprazolam	12	0.25 mg to 0.5 mg
	Temazepam	8-12	10mg to 20 mg
Short-acting (more lipophilic)	Triazolam	2-3	0.125mg to 0.25mg

Adverse effects:

- **Dependence**: If high doses are given for long periods of time, physical and psychological dependence may develop. Abrupt discontinuation can result in withdrawal symptoms such as anxiety, insomnia, and, in some cases, seizures. The risk is higher with short-acting drugs such as triazolam.

- Other side effects include drowsiness and confusion, the two most common side effects of the benzodiazepines, ataxia at high doses, and cognitive impairment.

Indications:

- Treatment of anxiety disorders including panic disorders, social anxiety disorders, post-traumatic stress disorders, and phobias. Benzodiazepines should not be routinely prescribed to alleviate the normal stress of day-to-day living. Because of their addictive nature, they should only be used for short periods of time to mitigate continued severe anxiety.

- Treatment of anxiety related to other mental health conditions, including depression and schizophrenia.

- Treatment of sleep disorders, including insomnia.

- Conscious sedation and amnesia during minor interventions such as endoscopy, or dental procedures.

- Treatment of seizures: Diazepam is the drug of choice for termination of status epilepticus.

- Treatment of muscle spasms in muscular disorders such as cerebral palsy and multiple sclerosis. They may also be used for muscle relaxation following muscle strains.

- Treatment of epilepsy.

Contraindications:

- Patients who are alcoholics, or are taking other CNS depressants: action can be potentiated.

- Patients with liver disease

- Pregnant women and breastfeeding mothers

- Patients with acute narrow-angle glaucoma

Benzodiazepine Antagonist

- Flumazenil is a specific antagonist for benzodiazepines. It competes with the drug for the GABA receptor and inhibits GABA action.

- The drug can only be administered intravenously, and it has a rapid onset of action.

- Flumazenil has a short half-life of one hour. Therefore, it is used to reverse toxicity of long- acting benzodiazepines. Multiple doses may be needed to maintain reversal.

- Flumazenil can precipitate withdrawal symptoms in dependent patients, or cause seizures, particularly if the benzodiazepine was used to control seizure activity.

BARBITURATES

Barbiturates have largely been replaced today by benzodiazepines because of their potential to cause tolerance, physical dependence, and severe withdrawal symptoms. However, they were once the most commonly used sedative-hypnotic drugs.

Mechanism of action:

Like benzodiazepines, barbiturates target GABA receptors to potentiate the inhibitory effect of GABA. The binding site on the receptor is distinct from the binding site of benzodiazepines. Barbiturates also bind to glutamate receptors, and inhibit glutamate, which is an excitatory neurotransmitter. In addition to this, certain barbiturates (like pentobarbital) block sodium channels which enhances the inhibitory effect.

Clinical effects:

- **CNS depression** : Barbiturates cause CNS depression in a dose-dependent manner. At low doses, they have a sedative effect. At slightly higher doses, they act as hypnotics. At still higher doses, they can cause anesthesia, and, at toxic doses, can result in coma and death.

- **Respiratory depression** : Barbiturates block chemoreceptor and hypoxic-mediated response to carbon dioxide, leading to respiratory depression.

Pharmacokinetics:

- Oral route of administration; Absorbed from the gut and sent to the CNS.
- From the CNS, it redistributes rapidly to the skeletal muscles and adipose tissue.
- Metabolism in the liver, excreted in urine.
- Barbiturates can cross the placental barrier and cause CNS and respiratory depression in the fetus.

Adverse effects:

- Drowsiness, sluggishness, and impaired ability to concentrate.
- Withdrawal symptoms can be severe and include anxiety, restlessness, tremors, seizures, and delirium.
- Barbiturates diminish the action of drugs which are metabolized through the cytochrome P450 system.
- Drug hangover leading to impaired functioning for several hours after the patient wakes up.
- Barbiturate poisoning due to overdosage.

Indications:

- **Anesthesia** : Thiopental, an ultrashort-acting barbiturate, has been used as an induction agent in general anesthesia.
- **Anti-epileptic** : Phenobarbital has been used for treatment of status epilepticus, as well as for long-term seizure management.
- **Treatment of anxiety and insomnia** : They have largely been replaced by benzodiazepines, because of their adverse effects.

Contraindications:

- Patients with acute intermittent porphyria
- Pregnant women

OTHER (NON-BENZODIAZEPINE) ANXIOLYTICS

Zolpidem

- Although it is structurally unrelated to benzodiazepines, its mechanism of action is similar. It binds to the benzodiazepine binding site on the receptor and potentiates GABA.
- It only produces a hypnotic effect. It does not have anti-epileptic or muscle relaxing properties.
- It is usually absorbed from the oral route, but sublingual preparations are also available. It has a fast onset of action of 30 minutes. T1/2 is 2 to 3 hours, but the clinical effect lasts for five hours.
- It is metabolized by hepatic oxidation (CYP450 system).
- Zolpidem can cause anterograde amnesia, daytime drowsiness, agitation, dizziness, and headaches.

Zaleplon

- It is similar to zolpidem with regard to mechanism of action.
- It has a similar onset of action, but shorter half-life (one hour). Clinical effects last for three hours. This drug has fewer side effects than zolpidem.
- Metabolism occurs in the liver through the CYP3A4 enzyme

Zopiclone:

- This was the first non-Benzodiazepine anxiolytic to be introduced, and is not much in use today.
- It has a similar mechanism of action and parmacokinetics as the above drugs. Its t1/2 is 5-6 hours
- Adverse effects include bitter taste, dry mouth and psychological disturbances.
- Indications: Usually used when weaning off from benzodiazepines.

EXERCISES

1. Which of the following drugs does not bind to the benzodiazepine binding site of the GABA receptor?
   a. Diazepam
   b. Zolpidem
   c. Triazolam
   d. Thiopental

2. Which of the following is not a therapeutic use of diazepam?
   a. Treatment of anxiety disorders
   b. Treatment of status epilepticus
   c. Treatment of schizophrenia
   d. Treatment of muscle spasm in cerebral palsy

3. Which of the following is a long-acting benzodiazepine?
   a. Diazepam
   b. Triazolam
   c. Alprazolam
   d. Temazepam

4. Which of the following is a specific antagonist for benzodiazepines?
   a. Flurazepam
   b. Flumazenil
   c. Fluconazole
   d. Fluoxetine

5. Which of the following drugs is contraindicated in patients with acute intermittent porphyria?
   a. Diazepam
   b. Zolpidem
   c. Phenobarbital
   d. Alprazolam

6. What is the half-life of alprazolam?
   a. 6 hours
   b. 8 hours
   c. 12 hours
   d. 16 hours

7. What is the correct dosage of triazolam?
   a. 0.125 to 0.25 mg
   b. 0.25 to 0.5 mg
   c. 1 to 2 mg
   d. 10 mg

8. How do barbiturates affect drugs metabolized through the P450 system?
   a. Enhance activity
   b. Diminish activity
   c. Enhance some and diminish some drugs
   d. No effect

9. What kind of amnesia is produced by benzodiazepines?
   a. Retrograde amnesia
   b. Anterograde amnesia
   c. Complete amnesia
   d. No amnesia

10. Which of the following clinical effects is produced by zolpidem?
    a. Muscle relaxation
    b. Analgesia
    c. Hypnotic
    d. Anti-epileptic

CHAPTER 3

Opioid Analgesics

The most common reason that patients seek medical treatment is pain. Acute pain is largely managed by the use of non-steroidal anti-inflammatory drugs (NSAIDS), which will be dealt with in a subsequent chapter. However, NSAIDS are not suitable for the management of chronic pain, because of the undesirable effects associated with long-term use. Moreover, NSAIDS are ineffective in severe pain syndromes, such as pain in malignancy. In these situations, opioid analgesics are the preferred agents for pain management.

The body produces endogenous opioids, such as endorphins and enkephalins. These opioids function as inhibitory neurotransmitters, and prevent the pain impulse from being transmitted from the spinal cord to the brain. Therapeutic opioids are similar to these compounds.

MECHANISM OF ACTION

Opioids bind to three receptor sites on the neuronal surface – the μ, κ, and δ receptors. These are G-protein-coupled receptors, and, when the drug binds to the receptor, there is inhibition of adenylyl cyclase. Drug binding also causes an influx of calcium ions in the presynaptic region, which impedes neuronal firing, and efflux of potassium ions in the postsynaptic region, which causes hyper-polarization of the neuron. All these factors help in attenuation of the pain impulse at a central level, bringing about relief from pain.

Based on their interaction with the opioid receptor, there are three classes of drugs – full opioid agonists, partial opioid agonists, and opioid antagonists.

OPIOID AGONISTS

Types of opioid analgesics:

Based on their origin, opioids may be classified as natural, semi-synthetic, or synthetic drugs. These drugs can also be classified based on their chemical structure (Table 1).

Table 1. Classification of opioids based on their chemical structure

PHENANTHRENE	BENZMORPHAN	PHENYLPIPERIDINES	DIPHENYLHEPTANES
Morphine	Pentazocine	Fentanyl	Methadone
Codeine		Meperidine	
Oxycodone			

Clinical effects:

- **Effects on the central nervous system** : Opioids have three effects on the CNS.
  - o Analgesia: Opioid analgesics attenuate nerve impulses at the spinal cord level. Some opioids, like morphine, also alter the brain's perception of pain, bringing further pain relief. Codeine is a relatively weak analgesic. Oxycodone is twice as potent as morphine when given orally, while oxymorphone is three times as potent orally. Oral hydromorphone is 8 to 10 times more potent than morphine.
  - o Euphoria: Opioids, morphine in particular, induce a calming effect and can produce a sense of extreme well-being and contentment.
  - o Sedation: In larger doses, some opioids have a sedative effect. Sedation is dose-dependent and progressively higher doses can cause unconsciousness and coma.
- **Respiratory effects** : Some opioids such as morphine depress the sensitivity of the respiratory center to carbon dioxide. This respiratory depression is the leading cause of death due to opioid overdose. However, tolerance develops with repeated doses. Morphine and codeine also suppress the cough center. Morphine causes histamine release from mast cells, which can cause bronchoconstriction.
- **Ophthalmic effects** : Morphine causes pupillary miosis.
- **GI effects** : Morphine stimulates the chemoreceptor trigger zone for emesis and may cause vomiting. It increases muscle tone in the intestinal smooth muscles and anal sphincter, and decreases GI motility. This leads to constipation.
- **Cardiovascular effects** : At larger doses, opioids can cause hypotension and bradycardia.

Contraindications:

- Severe brain injury
- Asthmatics
- Liver failure

Pharmacokinetics:

- Morphine is usually administered parenterally because it undergoes high first-pass metabolism. The other opioids are given as oral preparations.

- Morphine enters most body tissues, and can cross the placenta. It is not lipophilic and therefore does not cross the blood-brain barrier.

- Opioids usually undergo metabolism in the liver. Most opioids are metabolized by the cytochrome P450 system. Morphine, however, undergoes conjugation reaction. Some of the metabolites are also clinically effective. For instance, morphine is conjugated to morphine 6-glucuronide, which is a potent analgesic.

- Excretion primarily occurs through urine.

Adverse effects:

- **Respiratory depression** : This is most common with morphine, and patients with emphysema or cor pulmonale are at high risk.

- **Dependence** : Chronic use can produce physical and psychological dependence.

PARTIAL AGONISTS AND MIXED AGONISTS-ANTAGONISTS

When partial agonists bind to the opioid receptor, they do not activate the receptors completely. Mixed agonist-antagonists can stimulate one receptor, but block others. When these drugs are used in opioid-naïve individuals (those who have not received opioids before), they act similar to opioids, and can produce analgesia. In patients who are opioid-tolerant, they may show blocking or antagonist effects. Some important drugs in this category are as follows:

Buprenorphine:

- Used through parenteral, sublingual, or transdermal route. It is metabolized in the liver and excreted through bile and urine.

- This has an analgesic effect that lasts for 6-8 hours, but does not cause respiratory depression, hypotension, or sedation

- This is used in opioid detoxification.

Pentazocine:

- It is administered orally or parenterally.

- Produces moderate analgesia, but less euphoria.

- It can cause respiratory depression and constipation at higher doses. It increases blood pressure, including systemic and pulmonary arterial pressure. It should therefore be avoided in patients with coronary artery disease.

OPIOID ANTAGONISTS

These drugs bind to the opioid receptors but do not activate them. They do not have any effect in opioid-naïve individuals. However, they reverse the effects of opioids in patients who have consumed them. They are therefore useful in managing drug overdose. The two important opioid antagonists are:

Naloxone:

- This is mainly used in morphine overdose. Injected intravenously, it acts within 30 seconds to reverse respiratory depression and coma
- Its half-life is 30 to 81 minutes. Therefore, doses may need to be repeated until opioids have been eliminated from the system.

Naltrexone:

- This has a longer duration of action, which lasts for up to 24 hours. It may be given orally.

—————————— EXERCISES ——————————

1. Which of the following is not a clinical effect of morphine?
    a. Constipation
    b. Suppression of cough center
    c. Mydriasis
    d. Bradycardia

2. Which of the following opioids has the most potent analgesic effect?
    a. Morphine
    b. Oxycodone
    c. Hydromorphone
    d. Oxymorphone

3. Which of the following drugs is preferred for opioid detoxification?
    a. Codeine
    b. Naltrexone
    c. Buprenorphine
    d. Pentazocine

4. Apart from morphine, which of the following opioids exhibits antitussive activity?
    a. Oxycodone
    b. Buprenorphine
    c. Codeine
    d. Pentazocine

5. Which of the following drugs is used as an emergency treatment for morphine overdose?
    a. Methadone
    b. Buprenorphine
    c. Fentanyl
    d. Naloxone

6. Which of the following is not an opioid receptor?
   a. μ
   b. γ
   c. δ
   d. κ

7. Why does morphine cause bronchoconstriction?
   a. Serotonin release
   b. Histamine release
   c. Prostaglandin release
   d. Adrenaline release

8. Which of the following opioids is a partial agonist?
   a. Methadone
   b. Buprenorphine
   c. Codeine
   d. Oxymorphone

9. In which category of patients should pentazocine be avoided?
   a. Asthmatics
   b. Patients with emphysema
   c. Patients with cardiovascular disease
   d. Patients with malignancy

10. What is the cause of death in morphine overdose?
   a. Myocardial infarction
   b. Respiratory depression
   c. Cardiac arrest
   d. Pulmonary embolism

CHAPTER 4

Antidepressants and Anti-Manic Drugs

Depression is simply defined as a state of sadness. In more complex terms, depression is a psychoneurotic disorder characterized by feelings of sadness or grief, difficulty in thinking and concentration, and a decline in mental and sometimes physical activity. Antidepressants, or mood elevators, are drugs that are used to treat depressive disorders.

Depressive disorders may either be unipolar or bipolar. Unipolar disorders are associated chiefly with depression. However, in bipolar disorders, bouts of depression alternate with bouts of mania (or excitation).

MECHANISM OF ACTION OF ANTIDEPRESSANTS:

The mechanism of action of antidepressants is based on the 'amine theory' of depression. The theory states that depression is caused by a functional deficiency of neurotransmitters, especially norepinephrine. Neurotransmitters serve as communicators between different neurons in the brain. They are released from the axons of one neuron, and are taken up by another neuron (re-uptake) once the transmission function is complete. Most antidepressants work by inhibiting reuptake of the neurotransmitter. This increases the concentration of the neurotransmitter in the extracellular fluid around the neurons.

Five key categories of drugs are used in the management of depressive disorders:

- Selective serotonin re-uptake inhibitors (SSRIs)
- Serotonin/ norepinephrine re-uptake inhibitors (SNRIS)
- Monoamine oxidase inhibitors (MAOIs)
- Tricyclic antidepressants (TCAs)
- Atypical antidepressants

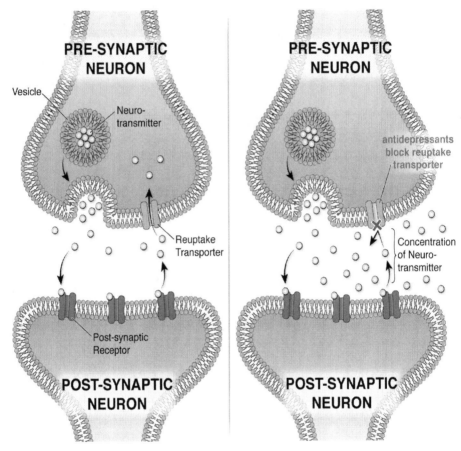

Figure 5 Amine theory states that depression is caused by a deficiency of neurotransmitters. Neurotransmitters are released from the axons of one neuron and are taken up (reuptake) by another neuron. Most antidepressants work by inhibiting reuptake, thereby increasing the concentration of neurotransmitter in the extracellular fluid around the neurons.

SELECTIVE SEROTONIN RE-UPTAKE INHIBITORS

SSRIs are the first-line drugs used in treatment of depression. These drugs have minimal side effects as compared to the other classes of drugs. These drugs block the re-uptake of serotonin, increasing its concentration at the neuronal synapse.

Pharmacokinetics:

- Route of administration is oral. Some SSRIs, like sertraline, have increased absorption if taken along with food.

- Most SSRIs have a plasma half-life between 16 to 36 hours. Fluoxetine alone has a longer half-life of 50 hours.

- Metabolism usually occurs in the liver, through the cytochrome P450 system and through conjugation by glucuronides and sulfates. However, some SSRIs like fluoxetine and paroxetine inhibit the CYP2D6 component of the P450 system.

ADVERSE EFFECTS:

- **Minor adverse effects** : SSRIs have minor adverse effects, including nausea, anxiety, sleep disturbances (both drowsiness and insomnia), and sexual dysfunction.

- **Overdose** : One SSRI, citalopram, can cause cardiac arrhythmias if overdose is taken. Other SSRIs are relatively safe even in overdose. If taken with an MAOI, all SSRIs can cause a serotonin syndrome manifested as hyperthermia, muscle rigidity, myoclonus, and alterations in vital signs and mental status.

- **Discontinuation syndrome** : If stopped abruptly, SSRIs can cause headache, flu-like symptoms, irritability, and sleep disturbances.

SEROTONIN/NOREPINEPHRINE RE-UPTAKE INHIBITORS

These drugs act by preventing the re-uptake of both serotonin as well as noradrenaline. The drug venlafaxine primarily inhibits serotonin, and, at larger doses, inhibits noradrenaline. On the other hand, duloxetine inhibits both serotonin and noradrenaline at all doses. They are therefore more effective than SSRIs. SNRIs have two main therapeutic applications:

- Treating depression in cases where SSRIs have proven ineffective
- Treating depression-associated chronic pain, such as backaches and muscle pain

Pharmacokinetics:

- All SNRIs are taken orally.
- They are metabolized by the cytochrome P450 system. Duloxetine may inhibit CYP2D6 isozymes. Duloxetine has maximum liver metabolism, and should be avoided in patients with liver disease.

Adverse effects:

- **Minor effects** : Nausea, headache, constipation, sexual dysfunction, dizziness, and sleep disturbances.
- Discontinuation syndrome may be seen similar to SSRIs.

TRICYCLIC ANTIDEPRESSANTS

Tricyclic antidepressants were the earlier first-line drugs used in depression. They have largely been replaced by SSRIs now because of their multiple side effects.

Mechanism of action:

- Most TCAs block re-uptake of both serotonin and noradrenaline into the presynaptic terminal. Some TCAs like maprotiline and desipramine selectively prevent only noradrenaline re-uptake.
- TCAs also block other receptors, including histaminic, muscarinic, α-adrenergic, and serotonergic receptors. This activity is largely responsible for the adverse effects of the TCAs.

Pharmacokinetics:

- Route of administration is oral. Bioavailability is unpredictable due to high first-pass metabolism.
- TCAs are lipophilic, and can easily penetrate the CNS.
- Metabolism occurs in the liver through the cytochrome P450 system as well as conjugation.
- Excreted in urine as inactive metabolites.

Therapeutic effects:

- **Treatment of moderate-to-severe depression** : TCAs improve mood and mental alertness, and even increase physical activity.
- **Treatment of bed-wetting** : Imipramine has been used to control bed-wetting in children older than six years of age.
- **Chronic pain syndromes** : Amitriptyline has been used for migraines and other chronic pain syndromes.
- **Insomnia** : Doxepin, in low doses, has been used for insomnia.

Adverse effects:

- **Muscarinic receptors blockade** : Xerostomia, blurred vision, constipation, urinary retention. They can cause sinus tachycardia, and, in overdoses, can cause arrhythmias.
- **α-adrenergic receptors blockade** : Orthostatic hypotension, reflex tachycardia.
- **Histamine receptors blockade** : Sedation, weight gain.

MONOAMINE OXIDASE INHIBITORS

Monoamine oxidase is a mitochondrial enzyme that serves to deactivate excess neurotransmitters (including noradrenaline, serotonin, and dopamine). MAOIs inhibit this enzyme, causing the neurotransmitters to accumulate in the synaptic space. Most MAOIs cause irreversible inactivation, by forming stable complexes with the enzyme.

Therapeutic uses : MAOIs are used in depression that is unresponsive to SSRIs and TCAs. Atypical depression may be responsive only to MAOIs.

Pharmacokinetics:

They are well absorbed after oral administration. Although MAO is fully inhibited within a few days, the antidepressant action takes several weeks. The drug is metabolized in the liver and excreted through urine. Upon discontinuation, regeneration of MAO enzyme takes several weeks.

Adverse effects : MAOIs inhibit monoamine oxidase activity not only in the brain, but also in the gut and liver. This prevents oxidative deamination of drugs and toxins, which can lead to dangerous side effects. For instance, MAO catalyzes the degradation of dietary tyramine. With MAOIs, the accumulated tyramine can cause release of large amounts of catecholamines, which may lead to hypertensive crisis. This presents with hypertension, cardiac arrhythmias, seizures, occipital headache, and even stroke. Selegiline may avoid first-pass metabolism if administered as a transdermal patch, and may be used as a safer alternative.

ATYPICAL ANTIDEPRESSANTS

These are a mixed group of drugs which have different mechanisms of action. Some of the more important drugs in this category are as follows:

Bupropion:
* This drug inhibits re-uptake of dopamine and norepinephrine.
* **Adverse effects** : It does not cause sexual dysfunction. May cause dry mouth, sweating, nervousness, and tremors. Seizures may occur, and this is dose-dependent.
* This drug is used for managing withdrawal symptoms related to nicotine in patients who are quitting smoking.

Mirtazapine:
* This drug acts at the presynaptic α-2 adrenergic receptors and serotonergic receptors. It enhances the activity of both noradrenaline and serotonin.
* It can cause sedation, increased appetite, and weight gain

Trazodone and Nefazodone:
* These drugs weakly inhibit serotonin re-uptake.
* They are weakly sedating, and are also used to manage insomnia.

ANTI-MANIA DRUGS

Anti-mania drugs, or mood stabilizers, are primarily used in the treatment of bipolar depressive disorder. These drugs help prevent mood swings and may be employed for treatment of both depression and mania.

Lithium salts

The exact mechanism of action of lithium is unknown. Some authors believe that it replaces intracellular and extracellular sodium, while others believe that it selectively inhibits dopamine and noradrenaline, with no effect on serotonin.

Clinical effects:

- It does not have any effect in normal patients. However, in patients with bipolar disorder, it stabilizes the mood within 2 to 3 weeks.
- It inhibits the action of anti-diuretic hormone in the kidney, and may cause diabetes insipidus.
- It inhibits the release of thyroid hormones, and has an insulin-like effect on glucose metabolism.
- It may decrease leukocyte count.

Pharmacokinetics:

- It is well absorbed orally.
- It does not bind to plasma or tissue proteins. It enters the extracellular fluid first before being taken up by cells.
- It does not undergo any metabolism, and is excreted by the kidney in a manner similar to sodium ions.

Adverse effects:

- **Minor adverse effects** : Headache, dry mouth, polyuria, polyphagia, polydipsia, sedation, and dermatological reactions.

OTHER ANTI-MANIA DRUGS

Other classes of CNS drugs are used for treatment of mania. They are described in detail in the appropriate sections. These drugs include:

- **Antiepileptic drugs** : Carbamazepine, sodium valproate, lamotrigine.
- **Neuroleptics and newer antipsychotic drugs** : Chlorpromazine, haloperidol, risperidone etc.

EXERCISES

1. Which of the following drugs does not inhibit noradrenaline reuptake?
   a. Amitriptyline
   b. Desipramine
   c. Duloxetine
   d. Sertraline

2. Which of the following SSRIs has the longest duration of action?
   a. Paroxetine
   b. Fluoxetine
   c. Sertraline
   d. Citalopram

3. Which of the following classes of antidepressants are the safest to use as first-line treatment in depression?
   a. Selective serotonin reuptake inhibitors
   b. Serotonin norepinephrine reuptake inhibitors
   c. Tricyclic antidepressants
   d. Monoamine oxidase inhibitors

4. Which of the following drugs are used for treatment of typical depression?
   a. Selective serotonin reuptake inhibitors
   b. Serotonin norepinephrine reuptake inhibitors
   c. Tricyclic antidepressants
   d. Monoamine oxidase inhibitors

5. Which of the following is not used in the management of mania?
   a. Lithium
   b. Carbamazepine
   c. Sertraline
   d. Chlorpromazine

6. Which of the following classes of antidepressants has the maximum adverse effects?
   a. SSRIs
   b. SNRIs
   c. TCAs
   d. MAOIs

7. Mechanism of action of antidepressants is based on which theory?
   a. Oxidation theory
   b. Amine theory
   c. Glucuronide theory
   d. Catecholamine theory

8. How is lithium metabolized in the body?
   a. Oxidation
   b. Hydrolysis
   c. Conjugation
   d. Does not get metabolized

9. What is the half-life of most SSRIs?
   a. 10-15 hours
   b. 16-36 hours
   c. 26-46 hours
   d. 40-50 hours

10. Which of the following is not an atypical antidepressant?
    a. Bupropion
    b. Mirtazapine
    c. Buprenorphine
    d. Trazodone

CHAPTER 5

Antipsychotics

Antipsychotics are a specific class of drugs that are primarily used in the treatment of schizophrenia. However, these drugs may also be applied to the treatment of mania, and other psychotic disorders.

Antipsychotic drugs work on the 'dopamine hypothesis' of psychotic disorders. According to this hypothesis, psychotic disorders such as schizophrenia occur due to dysregulation of dopamine in the neurological pathways of the brain. Specifically, there is hyperactivity of dopamine in the mesolimbic area, while other areas, such as mesocortical area, tuberoinfundibular area, and nigrostriatal area show hypoactivity.

MECHANISM OF ACTION OF ANTIPSYCHOTIC DRUGS:

Based on their mechanism of action, these drugs have been classified into first generation and second generation antipsychotics (Table 1).

First generation drugs act by competitively blocking dopamine D2 receptors of all the neuronal pathways apart from the mesolimbic area. Therefore, functioning of other areas where dopamine hypoactivity may be present (like the mesocortical area) may be worsened. The high potency drugs in this category block only D2 receptors, however, low potency drugs may also block the α-adrenergic, cholinergic, and histamine receptors

The second generation antipsychotics (also called atypical antipsychotics) block dopamine D2 receptors, as well as serotonin 5HT-2A receptors. The D2 receptor blockade is temporary, unlike first generation drugs. Since serotonin inhibits dopamine, and these drugs inhibit serotonin, they basically cause an increase in dopamine levels at certain areas of the brain. So, areas like the mesocortical area may benefit from using these drugs over first generation drugs.

Table 1. Classification of antipsychotic drugs

FIRST GENERATION		SECOND GENERATION
HIGH POTENCY	**LOW POTENCY**	
Haloperidol Loxapine Pimozide Fluphenazine	Chlorpromazine Thioridazine Prochlorperazine	Aripiprazole Risperidone Clozapine Olanzapine Quetiapine

Clinical Effects:

- **CNS** : In normal individuals, these drugs can produce 'neurolept anesthesia'. The individual becomes indifferent to surroundings, and may go off to sleep, but is arousable. In individuals suffering from schizophrenia, these drugs can reduce hallucinations and delusions (mediated by hyperactivity of the mesolimbic pathway). However, the drugs also act on already hypoactive pathways, such as the mesocortical pathway, which mediates apathy and cognitive impairment. These symptoms do not resolve, and can even worsen.

- **Extrapyramidal effects** : These occur due to blockade of D2 receptors in the nigrostriatal pathway. This leads to dystonia, tremors, involuntary movements, and motor restlessness. This is less common with second generation drugs.

- **Endocrine effects** : Neuroleptic drugs can stimulate excess release of prolactin. This leads to gynecomastia and galactorrhea.

- **Antiemetic effects** : The drugs block D2 receptors in the chemoreceptor trigger zone (CTZ) in the medulla. This suppresses nausea.

- **Anticholinergic effects** : Some antipsychotics suppress the cholinergic receptors. This leads to dry mouth, blurred vision, constipation, and urinary retention.

- **Anti-adrenergic effects** : Blockade of α-adrenergic receptors can cause orthostatic hypotension.

Pharmacokinetics:

- Route of administration is mostly oral. The absorption of selected drugs, including ziprasidone and paliperidone is increased on intake with food.

- It has a large volume of distribution due to high degree of binding with both plasma and tissue proteins.

- Metabolism occurs in the liver through the CY-P450 system. The metabolites are often active, and many metabolites themselves have been developed for clinical use.

- Excretion occurs through the urine. The t1/2 of the drugs is highly variable. Half-life of the most common drugs is listed in Table 2.

Table 2. Half-life and dosage of common antipsychotics

CATEGORY	DRUG	HALF-LIFE	DOSE
FIRST GENERATION	Chlorpromazine	18-30 hours	100-800 mg/day
	Haloperidol	24 hours	2-20 mg/day
	Pimozide	48-60 hours	2-6 mg/day
SECOND GENERATION	Clozapine	12 hours	100-300 mg/day
	Olanzapine	24-30 hours	2.5-20 mg/day
	Quetiapine	6 hours	50-400 mg/day
	Ziprasidone	8 hours	40-160mg/day
	Aripiprazole	72 hours	5-30 mg/day

Adverse Effects:

- **Extrapyramidal effects** : These are mostly seen in first generation drugs.

- **Metabolic effects** : Some antipsychotics (olanzapine, clozapine) can increase glucose and triglyceride levels. They can precipitate or worsen diabetes.

- Other effects due to blockade of cholinergic and adrenergic receptors, and due to stimulation of prolactin – are mild but undesirable.

- **Neuroleptic malignant syndrome** : This sometimes develops with first generation high- potency drugs. The patient develops muscle rigidity, fever, myoglobinemia, and altered mental status. Treatment is supportive, and the antipsychotic must be discontinued.

Indications:

- Psychotic disorders, primarily schizophrenia
- Prevention of nausea and vomiting:
  - o Vertigo related: Meclizine
  - o Motion sickness: Promethazine
  - o Related to cancer chemotherapy: Haloperidol, Prochlorperazine

- Intractable hiccups: Chlorpromazine is usually used.

Contraindications:

Patients with seizure disorders – may precipitate seizures.

—————————————————— EXERCISES ——————————————————

1. Which neurotransmitter is dysregulated in psychotic disorders?
   a. Serotonin
   b. Dopamine
   c. Noradrenaline
   d. Acetylcholine

2. Which of the following drugs is not a high-potency drug?
   a. Pimozide
   b. Chlorpromazine
   c. Haloperidol
   d. Fluphenazine

3. Intake of which of the following drugs with food increases its absorption?
   a. Ziprasidone
   b. Fluphenazine
   c. Risperidone
   d. Olanzapine

4. Which of the following conditions may be precipitated with antipsychotics?
   a. Myocardial infarction
   b. Asthma
   c. Epilepsy
   d. Angina

5. Which of the following hormones undergoes increased production when antipsychotic drugs are given?
   a. Estrogen
   b. Prolactin
   c. Progesterone
   d. Testosterone

6. Which of the following areas of the brain becomes hyperactive in psychotic disorders?
   a. Nigrostriatal
   b. Tuberoinfundibular
   c. Mesocortical
   d. Mesolimbic

7. What is the half-life of aripiprazole?
   a. 12 hours
   b. 24 hours
   c. 48 hours
   d. 72 hours

8. Which drug is used to treat intractable hiccups?
   a. Prochlorperazine
   b. Chlorpromazine
   c. Haloperidol
   d. Fluphenazine

9. Which of the following drugs can precipitate hyperglycemia?
   a. Olanzapine
   b. Quetiapine
   c. Ziprasidone
   d. Aripiprazole

10. The extrapyramidal adverse effects are reduced in second generation drugs. This is due to blockade of which receptors?
    a. Serotonin
    b. Adrenergic
    c. Muscarinic
    d. Cholinergic

CHAPTER 6

Drugs Used in Neurodegenerative Diseases

Neurodegenerative diseases are conditions that are caused due to destruction and degeneration of neurons in the central nervous system. The most common neurodegenerative diseases include Parkinsonism and Alzheimer's.

PARKINSON'S DISEASE

Parkinsonism is a neurodegenerative disease that affects areas of the brain that control muscle movements. The two main areas of the brain that control muscle activity are the substantia nigra and the neostriatum. The substantia nigra sends signals to the neostriatum through release of dopamine from dopaminergic neurons. In Parkinson's, there is degeneration of these neurons, which results in a deficiency of dopamine. Within the neostriatum, dopamine tends to inhibit GABA and acetylcholine. In its absence, there is overproduction of acetylcholine, which causes abnormal signaling. This is ultimately responsible for the uncontrolled movements seen in Parkinsonism.

Strategy for therapy in Parkinsonism:

Drug therapy in Parkinsonism usually involves the use of multiple drugs. The different classes are as follows:

Drugs used to replenish dopamine levels:

The ideal drug to use would be dopamine itself. However, this is not practical as dopamine does not cross the blood-brain barrier. Therefore, a more feasible alternative is the use of levodopa (L-dopa), which is its precursor. L-dopa easily crosses the barrier, and once within the brain, may be metabolized to dopamine.

Clinical effects:

- **CNS** : Once converted to dopamine, L-dopa exerts its clinical effects by providing symptomatic improvements. There is a decrease in muscle rigidity and tremors. With continued therapy, even gait, speech, and facial expressions are improved.

- **CVS** : Peripherally converted dopamine acts on β-adrenergic receptors, leading to tachycardia and postural hypotension.
- **Others** : Stimulation of receptors at the CTZ can trigger nausea and vomiting. Stimulation of the pituitary causes prolactin release.

Pharmacokinetics

Oral route of administration. It is absorbed from the small intestine. Prior to entering the brain, this drug may be degraded by two key enzymes – DDC (Dopa decarboxylase) and COMT (Catechol-O Methyltransferase). This reduces the bioavailability of the active drug. Once within the brain, it gets converted by DDC to dopamine, through which it exerts its actions.

Within the brain, L-dopa may be degraded by COMT as well as MAO (Monoamine oxidase). The inactive metabolites undergo conjugation and are excreted in urine. The plasma half-life of the drug is usually 1-2 hours.

Adverse effects:
- Nausea and vomiting, altered taste sensation.
- Postural hypotension, tachycardia.
- Visual and auditory hallucinations, mood changes, anxiety, depression, psychosis.

Indications:
- Early stages of Parkinson's disease

Contraindications:
- Patients on MAO inhibitors: can precipitate hypertensive crisis.
- Patients with psychosis: symptoms may be exacerbated.
- Patients with heart disease: can precipitate arrhythmias and angina.

Drugs used to maximize the effects of L-dopa:

L-dopa undergoes metabolism outside the CNS before it can cross into the brain. Within the brain also, it can undergo fast degradation. Therefore, certain drugs are given along with L-dopa to prevent its metabolism and increase the clinical effect. Some of these drugs are listed below:

Carbidopa : Carbidopa inhibits DDC. This prevents the metabolism of L-dopa in the periphery. Carbidopa can reduce the dose of L-dopa by four to five times, which in turn reduces the severity of adverse effects. It cannot penetrate the blood-brain barrier, and therefore, has no effect on L-dopa in the brain.

Selegiline and Rasagiline : These drugs inhibit MAO type B, which is responsible for the degradation of dopamine in the brain. As a result, these drugs increase dopamine levels in the brain, and enhance the action of L-dopa. These drugs may cause hypertension in high doses. Selegiline is metabolized to amphetamines, and may cause insomnia if taken in the evening.

Entacapone and Tolcapone : These drugs inhibit COMT. They are taken orally, are readily absorbed, and bind to plasma albumin, which decreases their distribution. These drugs are metabolized in the liver, and excreted in both urine and feces. Tolcapone has a longer duration of action, but also has the potential to cause fulminant hepatic necrosis, so is not preferred. These drugs reduce the 'wearing off' effect that is seen with L-dopa.

Using dopaminergic drugs:

L-dopa is only effective in the early stages of the disease. In later stages, there is degeneration of dopaminergic neurons, so that dopamine can no longer be synthesized from L-dopa within the neuron. Therefore, instead of L-dopa, dopaminergic drugs may be used. These drugs are agonists of dopamine. They bind to the dopamine receptors and exert actions similar to dopamine. A few drugs in this category are as follows:

Bromocriptine:
- This is a potent D2 agonist.
- Side effects include hallucinations, confusion, delirium, vomiting, and orthostatic hypotension. It can also cause pulmonary and retroperitoneal fibrosis.

Pramipexole and ropinirole:
- These are agonists for D2 and D3 receptors.
- They may be taken orally. Pramipexole does not metabolize much, while ropinirole undergoes extensive hepatic metabolism. They are excreted in the urine.
- The drug half-life is 8 hours and 6 hours respectively.
- They may cause daytime sleepiness, hallucinations, and postural hypotension.
- Apomorphine and rotigotine are similar drugs, which are used in injectable and transdermal forms respectively.

Amantadine:
- This drug has multiple effects. It increases dopamine secretion, and also inhibits cholinergic and NMDA type of glutamate receptors.
- This is used for early stages of the disease, and, for advanced cases, may be used in combination with L-dopa.
- Side effects: it can cause restlessness, confusion, and hallucinations. It can also cause orthostatic hypotension, constipation, urinary retention, and dry mouth.

Use of anticholinergic drugs:

Another strategy of treatment is to inhibit the over-activity of acetylcholine. This is done by the use of anticholinergic drugs. Anticholinergic drugs are described in detail in Unit 3.

ALZHEIMER DISEASE

Alzheimer disease is another neurodegenerative disease, which is characterized by abnormal protein deposition in the brain. The protein may deposit as plaques (amyloid) or tangle (tau). This deposition affects neurotransmission, and levels of critical neurotransmitters, such as acetylcholine, are reduced. Over time, there is degeneration of cholinergic neurons. There also appears to be overstimulation of NMDA glutamate receptors, which is believed to accelerate the degenerative process. Treatment in Alzheimer's therefore has the following strategies:

Improving cholinergic transmission:

This is done by the use of drugs that inhibit the enzyme acetylcholinesterase (ACE inhibitors). Inhibition of ACE prevents degradation of acetylcholine, which increases its levels and improves cholinergic transmission. ACE inhibitors that are used for Alzheimer disease include galantamine, rivastigmine, and donepezil.

Inhibiting NMDA glutamate stimulation:

Memantine is an NMDA receptor antagonist. It binds to the receptor and prevents inflow of excessive amounts of calcium ions, which are responsible for cell apoptosis.

Both the above drug classes may produce short term benefits in improving symptoms. However, the treatment is largely palliative as the underlying degenerative process cannot be halted.

EXERCISES

1. What kind of neuron is associated with degeneration in Parkinson's disease?
   a. Cholinergic
   b. NMDA associated
   c. Dopaminergic
   d. Adrenergic

2. Which of the following enzymes is inhibited by carbidopa?
   a. Dopa decarboxylase
   b. Catechol O methyltransferase
   c. Monoamine oxidase A
   d. Monoamine oxidase B

3. Which of the following enzymes is inhibited by selegiline?
   a. Dopa decarboxylase
   b. Catechol O methyltransferase
   c. Monoamine oxidase A
   d. Monoamine oxidase B

4. Which of the following enzymes is inhibited by Entocapone?
   a. Dopa decarboxylase
   b. Catechol O methyltransferase
   c. Monoamine oxidase A
   d. Monoamine oxidase B

5. What is the half-life of Pramipexole?
   a. 6 hours
   b. 8 hours
   c. 10 hours
   d. 12 hours

6. Which dopaminergic drug can be combined with L-dopa in later stages of Parkinsonism?
   a. Bromocriptine
   b. Ropinirole
   c. Apomorphine
   d. Amantadine

7. Which of the following drugs reduces the peripheral adverse effects of L-dopa, including nausea, vomiting and postural hypotension?
   a. Selegiline
   b. Amantadine
   c. Carbidopa
   d. Entocapone

8. Which of the following drugs can cause fulminant hepatic necrosis?
   a. Selegiline
   b. Rasagiline
   c. Entocapone
   d. Tolcapone

9. Which of the following neurotransmitters is reduced in Alzheimer disease?
   a. Glutamate
   b. Acetylcholine
   c. Noradrenaline
   d. Dopamine

10. Which of the following drugs used for Alzheimer's works by blocking NMDA receptors?
    a. Galantamine
    b. Rivastigmine
    c. Donepezil
    d. Memantine

CHAPTER 7

Anti-Epileptic Drugs

Epilepsy, or seizure disorders, are a group of conditions that occur due to sudden, excessive, and synchronous discharge of cerebral neurons. The excessive electrical activity may manifest in several different ways, and based on this, there are two main types of seizures – focal seizures, which are restricted to a specific portion of the brain, and generalized seizures, which may affect both the hemispheres of the brain. A broader classification is given below:

FOCAL SEIZURES:

- **Simple partial**: Abnormal activity of a single group of muscles, or limb.
- **Complex partial**: Associated with altered consciousness or hallucinations. Abnormal motor movements include diarrhea, urination, and chewing.

GENERALIZED SEIZURES:

- **Tonic-clonic seizures**: Most common. Loss of consciousness followed by tonicity (continuous contraction) and clonicity (rapid contraction and relaxation) occuring in alternating phases.
- **Absence seizures**: Characterized by self-limiting loss of consciousness.
    - o **Clonic and myoclonic seizures**: Consist of episodes of muscle contractions.
    - o **Tonic seizures**: Consist of increased muscle tone.
    - o **Atonic seizures**: Reverse of tonic seizures; there is a sudden loss of muscle tone.
    - o **Status epilepticus**: A life-threatening condition characterized by a series of seizures without recovery of consciousness in between.

DRUGS USED FOR THE MANAGEMENT OF EPILEPSY:

The following classes of drugs are used in the treatment of epilepsy:

- **Hydantoin drugs** : Phenytoin, Fosphenytoin
- **Iminostilbenes** : Carbamazepine, Oxcarbazepine
- **Succinimide** : Ethosuximide
- **Aliphatic carboxylic acid** : Sodium valproate

- **Phenyltriazines** : Lamotrigine
- **Cyclic GABA analogues** : Gabapentin, Pregabalin
- **Benzodiazepines** : Diazepam, Clonazepam, Lorazepam
- **Barbiturates and deoxybarbiturates** : Phenobarbitone, Primidone
- **Miscellaneous drugs** : Topiramate, Vigabatrin

A few of the most commonly used anti-epileptic drugs are described in detail below.

HYDANTOIN DRUGS

Mechanism of action:

- Binding, and blockade of voltage-gated sodium channels.

Pharmacokinetics:

- Oral absorption is slow and bioavailability is poor because of high degree of plasma protein binding. It is metabolized in the liver by hydroxylation and glucuronide conjugation. Metabolites are excreted through urine. The liver enzymes have limited capacity to metabolize phenytoin. As a result, the half-life increases with an increase in dose. While the initial t1/2 may be 12-24 hours, it can increase to as much as 60 hours.

Adverse effects:

- Gingival hypertrophy: This occurs due to increase in collagen bundles of the gingiva.
- Hirsutism, acne, and coarsening of facial features.
- Osteomalacia: Phenytoin interferes with vitamin D activation.
- Megaloblastic anemia
- Fetal hydantoin syndrome: If used by pregnant women, phenytoin can cause cleft lip and palate, microcephaly, and other hypoplastic changes.

Indications:

- Focal seizures, generalized tonic-clonic seizures, status epilepticus.

Contraindications:

- Pregnant women.

CARBAMAZEPINE:

Mechanism of action:

- It prolongs the inactive state of voltage-gated sodium channels.

Pharmacokinetics:

- Oral absorption is poor, and it binds to plasma proteins. Metabolism occurs through oxidation, hydroxylation, and conjugation reactions. Unlike phenytoin, its t1/2 decreases over time due to auto-induction of metabolism. While the initial t1/2 is 20-40 hours, it can decrease to 10-20 hours over long-term use.

Adverse effects:

- Urinary retention and hyponatremia: Enhances the action of antidiuretic hormone.
- Dizziness, sedation, vertigo, ataxia.
- May cause hypersensitivity reactions including rashes, photosensitivity, and hepatitis.

Indications:

- Focal seizures, generalized tonic-clonic seizures.
- First choice drug for trigeminal neuralgia.
- Bipolar disorder.

Contraindications:

- Absence seizures – may enhance these seizures.

ETHOSUXIMIDE:

Mechanism of action:

- Inhibition of T-type calcium channels.

Pharmacokinetics:

- It is completely absorbed orally, does not bind to plasma proteins, and distributes well. Metabolism occurs in the liver through hydroxylation and glucuronide conjugation, and the drug is excreted through the urine. The plasma half-life ranges from 32 to 48 hours.

Adverse effects:

- Mood changes and agitation.
- Lack of concentration, headache, and drowsiness.

Indications:

- Absence seizures

SODIUM VALPROATE:

Mechanism of action:

- This works by multiple mechanisms, which include inhibition of GABA transaminase (an enzyme that degrades the inhibitory neurotransmitter GABA), blockade of sodium channels, as well as T-type calcium channels.

Pharmacokinetics:

- Good oral absorption, but binds to plasma proteins. Valproate is metabolized in the liver by oxidation and glucuronide conjugation, and is then excreted in the urine. It has a plasma half-life of 10-15 hours.

Adverse effects:

- Anorexia, vomiting, diarrhea
- Alopecia, weight gain
- Thrombocytopenia and bleeding tendencies.

Indications:

- Both focal and generalized seizures, including absence seizures.

Contraindications:

- Pregnancy – has been associated with neural tube defects.

LAMOTRIGINE:

Mechanism of action:

- Blocks voltage-gated sodium channels and prolongs sodium channel inactivation. It also blocks high voltage calcium channels.

Pharmacokinetics

- Well absorbed by oral route, metabolized in liver through glucuronide conjugation. Its plasma half-life is 24 hours. Concomitant valproate dosing may prolong its half-life as metabolism is inhibited.

Adverse effects:

- Dizziness, sleepiness, ataxia
- Vomiting

Indications:

- Focal seizures, all generalized seizures

GABAPENTIN:

Mechanism of action:

- Exact mechanism of action is unknown. However, it may interfere with voltage-dependent calcium channels.

Pharmacokinetics:

- Absorbed well through oral route, it does not undergo metabolism. It is excreted unchanged in urine. Plasma half-life is 6 hours.

Adverse effects:
- Dizziness, tiredness, sedation, and nystagmus.

Indications:
- Add-on drug for focal and generalized seizures
- Neuropathic pain
- Postherpetic pain

TOPIRAMATE:

Mechanism of action:
- It blocks voltage-gated sodium channels, and L-type calcium currents. It inhibits NMDA glutamate, and is a carbonic anhydrase inhibitor.

Pharmacokinetics:
- Similar to gabapentin, it is absorbed orally, does not metabolize, and is excreted unchanged in the urine. Its half-life is 24 hours.

Adverse effects:
- Impaired concentration, ataxia, poor memory, sedation
- Glaucoma, decreased sweating, hyperthermia
- Weight loss, renal stones

Indications:
- Focal seizures, generalized tonic-clonic and myoclonic seizures
- Prevention of migraine

EXERCISES

1. What is the first-line drug to be used in trigeminal neuralgia?
   a. Carbamazepine
   b. Topiramate
   c. Gabapentin
   d. Valproate

2. Which of the following drugs is not preferred for absence seizures?
   a. Carbamazepine
   b. Lamotrigine
   c. Ethosuximide
   d. Valproate

3. What is the half-life of gabapentin?
   a. 6 hours
   b. 10 hours
   c. 12 hours
   d. 16 hours

4. Which of the following channels are blocked when ethosuximide is used?
   a. Sodium channels
   b. T-type calcium channels
   c. L-type calcium channels
   d. Potassium channels

5. Which of the following drugs, if used during pregnancy, can cause the fetus to develop cleft lip?
   a. Topiramate
   b. Carbamazepine
   c. Valproate
   d. Phenytoin

6. Which of the following anticonvulsants can increase the half-life of lamotrigine?
    a. Topiramate
    b. Gabapentin
    c. Valproate
    d. Carbamazepine

7. Which of the following drugs does not undergo any metabolism?
    a. Gabapentin
    b. Carbamazepine
    c. Lamotrigine
    d. Phenytoin

8. Which drug is used for prevention of migraine?
    a. Topiramate
    b. Carbamazepine
    c. Lamotrigine
    d. Phenytoin

9. Which of the following drugs can enhance the action of antidiuretic hormone?
    a. Carbamazepine
    b. Lamotrigine
    c. Phenytoin
    d. Valproate

10. Which of the following drugs is preferred for non-specific neuropathic pain?
    a. Topiramate
    b. Gabapentin
    c. Lamotrigine
    d. Valproate

UNIT III : THE AUTONOMIC NERVOUS SYSTEM

CHAPTER 1

Cholinergic and Anticholinergic Drugs

INTRODUCTION TO THE AUTONOMIC NERVOUS SYSTEM

The nerves in our body form two main organized systems – the central nervous system, which consists of the brain and spinal cord, and the peripheral nervous system, which comprises all the nerves of the body.

The peripheral nervous system, again, is organized into two systems. The somatic nervous system deals with voluntary movements, while the autonomic system deals with vital functions and involuntary movements.

The autonomic nervous system, again, consists of two main components – the sympathetic nervous system and the parasympathetic nervous system.

Table 1. Highlights of sympathetic and parasympathetic nervous system

PROPERTY		SYMPATHETIC	PARASYMPATHETIC
Anatomical location		Thoracic and lumbar region of spinal cord	Cranial nerves 2,7,9,10 Sacral region of spinal cord
Length of axons	Presynaptic	Short	Long
	Postsynaptic	Long	Short
Neurotransmitter	Presynaptic	Acetylcholine	Acetylcholine
	Postsynaptic	Noradrenaline	Acetylcholine
Effect on body systems	Overall response	Fight or flight response	Rest and digest response
	Eyes	Pupillary dilation	Pupillary constriction
	Secretions	Inhibition of salivary secretion	Stimulation of salivary secretion
	Respiratory system	Relaxation of airway muscles - bronchodilation	Bronchoconstriction
	Cardiovascular system	Tachycardia	Bradycardia
	Digestive system	Inhibits digestion and gallbladder function Stimulated release of glucose from liver Relaxation of intestinal movements	Stimulates digestive activity and intestinal movement Stimulated glucose uptake by liver
	Endocrine system	Stimulates adrenal medulla to secrete epinephrine and norepinephrine	No effect
	Urinary system	Relaxation of bladder	Bladder contraction

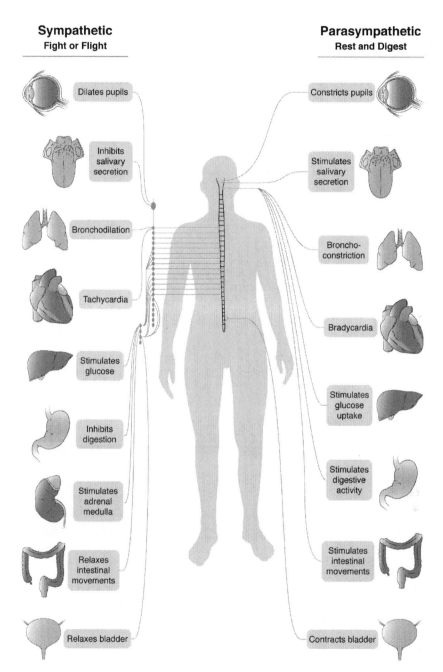

Sympathetic
Fight or Flight

Parasympathetic
Rest and Digest

Dilates pupils

Constricts pupils

Inhibits salivary secretion

Stimulates salivary secretion

Bronchodilation

Broncho-constriction

Tachycardia

Bradycardia

Stimulates glucose

Stimulates glucose uptake

Inhibits digestion

Stimulates digestive activity

Stimulates adrenal medulla

Relaxes intestinal movements

Stimulates intestinal movements

Relaxes bladder

Contracts bladder

Figure 6 The autonomic nervous system, responsible for vital functions and involuntary movements in the body, comprises the sympathetic and parasympathetic nervous systems.

RECEPTORS IN THE AUTONOMIC NERVOUS SYSTEM:

Nerve cells, or neurons interact with each other at a junction called synapse. The first neuron releases its neurotransmitter into the synaptic region. The neurotransmitter then attaches itself to the second neuron at a specific point on the cell membrane, referred to as the receptor. There are different kinds of receptors in the autonomic nervous system.

Receptors between the presynaptic and postsynaptic neurons in the brain/spinal cord:

Nicotinic receptors: These are common to both the sympathetic and parasympathetic nervous system. These are also called ionotropic receptors. When acetylcholine binds to these receptors, the ion channels open, facilitating influx of sodium and other ions. Nicotinic receptors are of two important subtypes – N_M and N_N. N_M receptors are found at the neuromuscular junction, while N_N receptors are found in the adrenal medulla and at autonomic ganglia.

Receptors between the postsynaptic neurons and the effector organs:

These are also called metabotropic receptors. When the neurotransmitter binds to these receptors, they activate second messengers, which then cause a cascade of events. This involves the presence of G-protein. These receptors are of two types:

Adrenergic receptors: These are located in the sympathetic nervous system, and are activated by adrenaline and noradrenaline. Adrenergic receptors are classified as α receptors and β receptors, and each of these have specific subtypes. Each subtype of adrenergic receptor is involved with specific sympathetic functions. These are detailed further in Chapter 2 of this unit.

Muscarinic receptors: These are located in the parasympathetic nervous system, and are activated by acetylcholine. This has five subtypes, named M1 to M5. Only M1 to M3 have been functionally characterized. M1 is located in the gastric glands, M2 in the heart, and M3 in the eyes, exocrine glands, lungs, and digestive tract.

CHOLINERGIC DRUGS

These are drugs that act at the cholinergic receptors. Based on the mechanism of action, they are classified into four subtypes, which are summarized in Table 2.

Table 2. Classification of cholinergic drugs

DIRECTLY ACTING	INDIRECTLY ACTING REVERSIBLE DRUGS	INDIRECTLY ACTING IRREVERSIBLE DRUGS	DRUGS CAUSING REACTIVATION OF ACETYLCHOLINE ESTERASE
Acetylcholine	Physostigmine	Echothiophate	Pralidoxime
Carbachol	Neostigmine		
Bethanechol	Pyridostigmine		
Cevimeline	Edrophonium		
Nicotine	Rivastigmine		
Pilocarpine	Donepezil		
	Galantamine		

KINETICS OF ACETYLCHOLINE:

Acetylcholine acts as a neurotransmitter in two kinds of cholinergic neurons – nicotinic and muscarinic. The following steps outline its synthesis and action:

- Free choline from plasma is taken into the cell. It combines with Coenzyme A to form acetylcholine. The enzyme that catalyzes this reaction is choline acetyltransferase.
- Within the cell, acetylcholine is stored in vesicles.
- When the action potential arrives at the neuron, there is an influx of calcium ions into the cell. This causes fusion of the vesicle to the cell membrane, and the contents get expelled into the synaptic space.
- Acetylcholine from the synaptic space can undergo three courses of action:
  o Bind with receptors on the postsynaptic cell membrane, which is responsible for effector response.
  o Bind to receptors on the presynaptic membrane, which serves as negative feedback and prevents further release of acetylcholine.
  o Excess gets degraded by acetylcholinesterase into choline and acetate. The choline is recycled into the cell.

PHARMACOLOGICAL ACTIONS OF ACETYLCHOLINE:

Actions through muscarinic receptors:

- Heart: Effects are exerted through M2 receptors. Bradycardia occurs due to effect on SA node. Slowing of conduction may cause partial or complete heart block. There is a decrease in force of atrial contraction and to some extent, ventricular contraction, which may decrease cardiac output.

- Blood vessels: Effect on M3 receptors causes vasodilation. This can cause facial flushing and hypotension.
- Smooth muscle contraction: This is also exhibited through M3 receptors. There is an increase in tone and peristalsis of GIT, and evacuation of bowel. Increase in ureteric peristalsis and bladder contraction causes voiding of urine. Contraction of bronchial smooth muscles can cause spasm and dyspnea.
- Secretory activity: Parasympathetically innervated glands are stimulated (M3 receptors) leading to increased salivation, sweat, and tears.
- Eye: Pupillary constriction occurs. Ciliary muscle contraction can increase outflow and reduce intraocular tension. This is beneficial in glaucoma.

Actions through nicotinic receptors:
- There is stimulation of both sympathetic and parasympathetic autonomic ganglia.
- Skeletal muscle contraction

Directly acting cholinergic drugs:
These drugs bind to cholinergic receptors and mimic the actions of acetylcholine. Based on the receptors with which they interact, they produce specific pharmacological effects. The drugs and their effects are summarized in Table 3.

Table 3. Summary of directly acting cholinergic drugs

DRUG	RECEPTOR STIMULATED	CLINICAL EFFECTS	THERAPEUTIC APPLICATIONS
Bethanechol	M3	Stimulates intestinal tone and peristalsis. Increases bladder tone and ureter peristalsis	Non-obstructive urinary retention. Neurological atony. Megacolon
Carbachol	M2, M3, N_n	Releases adrenaline from adrenal medulla. Both stimulation and depression of cardiac, GI systems.	Topically only - in the eye to treat glaucoma
Pilocarpine	M3	Miosis, stimulation of sweat, tears and saliva.	Xerostomia. Emergency reduction of intraocular pressure
Cevimeline	M3	Salivary stimulation	Xerostomia

INDIRECTLY ACTING REVERSIBLE CHOLINE AGONISTS:

These drugs are also known as anticholinesterase agents. They inhibit the enzyme acetylcholine esterase, and prevent the breakdown of acetylcholine. This increases the levels of acetylcholine in the synaptic region, and enhances its action. Some important drugs in this class are discussed below:

Edrophonium:
- This is a short-acting agent.
- It is absorbed and eliminated in urine rapidly. The duration of action lasts between 10 to 20 minutes.
- It is primarily used for diagnosis of myasthenia gravis. In MG, antibodies destroy the nicotinic receptors. Edrophonium boosts acetylcholine availability to the remaining receptors, and increases muscle strength.

Physostigmine:
- This is an intermediate-acting agent, and duration of action lasts from 30 minutes to 2 hours.
- It is used for treatment of atonic conditions of the bladder and intestine.
- It is also used to reverse atropine toxicity.
- It may adversely cause bradycardia and decreased cardiac output.

Neostigmine:
- Like physostigmine, this has an intermediate duration of action.
- It has a greater effect on the skeletal muscles. It is therefore used for management of myasthenia gravis, and to stimulate the bladder and GIT.
- It is also used to reverse neuromuscular blockade that is given as a part of general anesthesia.
- It does not enter the brain and cannot be used to counteract central effects of atropine toxicity.

Rivastigmine, Donepezil, Galantamine:
- These are specifically used for the management of Alzheimer disease.
- These drugs boost the availability of acetylcholine to cholinergic neurons, which are deficient in this condition. However, they cannot halt disease progression.

INDIRECTLY ACTING IRREVERSIBLE CHOLINE AGONISTS:

These drugs bind covalently and irreversibly to acetylcholinesterase. This results in consistently high levels of acetylcholine. These drugs are highly toxic, and many were developed as 'nerve gases' for use in wartime. Pesticides, including malathion and parathion, belong to this category (this is clinically relevant in cases of poisoning). The only clinically useful drug in this category is echothiophate.

Echothiophate:
- It produces intense miosis, and increases outflow of aqueous humor.
- It is used topically for treatment of open-angle glaucoma. It has a long duration of action, lasting up to 100 hours.
- Side effects of the topical solution include development of cataract. It is not commonly used now.

Antidote: Pralidoxime:
- Toxicity of these drugs can be reversed using pralidoxime. This drug reactivates acetylcholinesterase, by breaking the bond between the drug and the enzyme.
- If the drug 'ages' (loses an alkyl group), pralidoxime is no longer effective. Different drugs age at different rates.
- It cannot penetrate the central nervous system, and therefore does not reverse CNS symptoms.
- Pralidoxime is not effective for reversible ACE inhibitors.

ANTICHOLINERGIC DRUGS

These drugs antagonize the actions of acetylcholine at its receptors. Based on the kind of receptors at which these drugs act, they can be divided into three categories:

- **Antimuscarinic agents** : They are also called parasympatholytics. They only antagonize muscarinic receptors, thus allowing unopposed sympathetic action (through adrenergic receptors).
- **Antinicotinic agents** : They are also called ganglionic blockers, and block the actions of both sympathetic and parasympathetic ganglia.
- **Neuromuscular blockers** : They are also called skeletal muscle relaxants. They block the action of acetylcholine at the neuromuscular junction of skeletal muscles, which also has nicotinic receptors.

ANTIMUSCARINIC AGENTS:

These drugs usually allow unopposed sympathetic activity. The only exception is the neurons innervating the salivary and sweat glands (which are cholinergic). Some important drugs in this category are detailed below:

ATROPINE:

This drug has a high affinity for muscarinic receptors.

Clinical effects:

- Eye: Mydriasis, cycloplegia, increased intraocular pressure
- GIT: Has an antispasmodic effect, decreases GI motility.
- Cardiovascular: Tachycardia is seen at high doses.
- Others: Decrease in sweat can cause increased body temperature. There is decreased salivary secretion, causing xerostomia.

Pharmacokinetics:

- It is readily absorbed and undergoes partial metabolism in the liver. Excretion is through urine and the drug half-life is about four hours.

Indications:

- Topically to induce mydriasis, for diagnosis of refractive errors
- Antispasmodic and antisecretory agent
- For treatment of bradycardia
- Antidote for organophosphate poisoning

Adverse effects:

- Dry mouth, blurred vision
- Urinary retention, constipation
- Restlessness, confusion, hallucinations, delirium

SCOPOLAMINE:

This has greater effects on the CNS as compared to atropine, and a longer duration of action. It blocks short-term memory. In small doses, it can cause sedation, but higher doses cause excitement and euphoria.

Clinical uses

- For prevention of motion sickness, and prevention of postoperative nausea and vomiting.

OTHER ANTIMUSCARINIC AGENTS:

Other antimuscarinic agents have been developed for specific therapeutic uses. These are summarized in Table 4.

Table 4. Uses of common antimuscarinic agents

DRUG	THERAPEUTIC BENEFIT
Ipratropium Tiotropium	Inhalational agents used to treat asthma and COPD
Oxybutynin (transdermal patch) Fesoterodine Darifenacin	Treatment of overactive urinary bladder
Tropicamide Cyclopentolate	To induce mydriasis and cycloplegia prior to checking for refractive errors in the eye. Tropicamide produces mydriasis for 6 hours, cyclopentolate for 24 hours.
Benztropine Trihexyphenidyl	Parkinson's disease, to manage extrapyramidal symptoms.

ANTINICOTINIC DRUGS (GANGLIONIC BLOCKERS)

These drugs basically block the entire output of the autonomic nervous system, as they act at the ganglionic level. These drugs are not used therapeutically.

NICOTINE:

- This drug is of clinical interest because it is a component of cigarette smoke, and is therefore widely used. This drug first causes stimulation, and then depression of all autonomic ganglia.
- It induces enhanced release of several neurotransmitters.
- Increased release of dopamine and noradrenaline can cause pleasure and appetite suppression.
- There is tachycardia and increase in blood pressure.
- Increase in secretions and peristalsis.
- At high doses, there is fall in secretions, peristalsis, and drop in blood pressure.

Neuromuscular blockers:

These drugs block the transmission of acetylcholine at the motor endplate of the neuromuscular junction. These drugs are categorized as nondepolarizing blockers and depolarizing blockers.

NONDEPOLARIZING BLOCKERS:

These are also called competitive blockers. These drugs compete with acetylcholine for the nicotinic receptors. However, they do not stimulate the receptors upon binding. At low doses, this binding prevents depolarization of the cell membrane and inhibits muscle contraction. At high doses these drugs inhibit the ion channels as well, which further weakens neuromuscular transmission.

Clinical effects

- These drugs cause muscle paralysis. Paralysis begins with small muscles of the face and eye, and progresses to muscles of the fingers and limbs, and then, the neck and trunk. The intercostal muscles and diaphragm are the last to be affected.

Pharmacokinetics:

- This is summarized in Table 5.

Table 5. Kinetics of nondepolarizing blockers

DRUG	ABSORPTION	ONSET/DURATION OF ACTION	METABOLISM	EXCRETION
Atracurium		2 min / 40 min	Degraded spontaneously in plasma by ester hydrolysis	--
Cisatracurium	Intravenous or intramuscular	3 min / 90 min		
Pancuronium		3 min / 86 min	No metabolism	Urine
Rocuronium		1 min / 43 min	Liver	Bile
Vecuronium		2 min / 44 min		

Adverse effects:

- Pancuronium – vagolytic, may cause tachycardia
- Atracurium – releases histamine and can provoke seizures

DEPOLARIZING BLOCKERS:

These agents act similar to acetylcholine, and work by depolarizing the muscle membrane. However, they are resistant to degradation by acetylcholinesterase, and therefore remain attached to the receptor for a long time, thus producing constant stimulation. This eventually results in a longer refractory period, during which the muscle remains paralyzed. The only clinically useful drug in this category is succinylcholine.

SUCCINYLCHOLINE:

Clinical effects:

- Causes brief muscle fasciculations, followed by flaccid paralysis. Paralysis occurs in one minute and lasts for 8 minutes.

Pharmacokinetics:

- After intravenous injection, it undergoes rapid redistribution. It is degraded in plasma by the enzyme pseudocholinesterase.

Adverse effects:

- Postoperative muscle pain
- Increased intraocular and intragastric pressure
- Potential for malignant hyperthermia
- Patients with an atypical form of pseudocholinesterase may develop prolonged apnoea.

--- EXERCISES ---

1. Which of the following is not an effect of the sympathetic nervous system?
   a. Miosis
   b. Mydriasis
   c. Increased bladder tone
   d. Bronchodilation

2. What kind of neurotransmitter is seen at the neuro-effector junction of the sympathetic nervous system?
   a. Noradrenaline
   b. Dopamine
   c. Acetylcholine
   d. Serotonin

3. What neurotransmitter is seen at the nicotinic receptors?
   a. Noradrenaline
   b. Dopamine
   c. Acetylcholine
   d. Serotonin

4. Which muscarinic receptor is involved with regulation of cardiac activity?
   a. M1
   b. M2
   c. M3
   d. M4

5. Which of the following drugs is used to reverse neuromuscular block following general anesthesia?
   a. Physostigmine
   b. Neostigmine
   c. Rivastigmine
   d. Pyridostigmine

6. How does Rivastigmine provide symptom relief in Alzheimer's disease?

a. Decreases neurological tangles
b. Dissolves amyloid plaques
c. Increases acetylcholine levels available for the existing receptors
d. Prevents degradation of cholinergic neurons

7. Which drug is used as a diagnostic agent for myasthenia gravis?
a. Edrophonium
b. Echothiophate
c. Physostigmine
d. Neostigmine

8. Which of the following drugs used for glaucoma has the longest duration of action?
a. Edrophonium
b. Echothiophate
c. Pilocarpine
d. Neostigmine

9. Which drug is preferred to induce mydriasis and cycloplegia, as it has the least duration of action?
a. Atropine
b. Pilocarpine
c. Tropicamide
d. Cyclopentolate

10. Which of the following neuromuscular blocker does not get degraded in plasma?
a. Vecuronium
b. Succinylcholine
c. Atracurium
d. Cisatracurium

CHAPTER 2

Adrenergic Agonists and Antagonists

The adrenergic receptors are located at the neuro-effector junction of the sympathetic nervous system. They are also located on the surface of the adrenal medulla.

ADRENERGIC AGONISTS

These are also known as adrenergic drugs, or sympathomimetic drugs. These drugs activate the adrenergic receptors either directly, or indirectly by increasing levels of norepinephrine available for binding to the receptors. They are classified as:

- **Directly acting agonists** : Like norepinephrine, they directly act at the receptor to produce similar actions. Examples include epinephrine, albuterol, salmeterol, isoproterenol, terbutaline, and phenylephrine.

- **Indirectly acting agonists** : They stimulate the release of norepinephrine, which enhances the clinical effect. Examples include cocaine and amphetamines.

- **Mixed action agonists** : They act both by interacting with the receptor, as well as by boosting the production of norepinephrine. Examples include ephedrine and pseudoephedrine.

Functions mediated by adrenergic receptors:

As stated in the previous chapter, each adrenergic receptor mediates specific sympathetic functions. These are summarized in Table 1.

Table 1. Functions of adrenergic receptors

RECEPTOR	α		β	
	α1	α2	β1	β2
METABOLIC EFFECT	Increases intracellular calcium ions	Decreases cAMP production	Activation of adenylyl cyclase, increased cAMP production	
CLINICAL EFFECT	Vasoconstriction Increased peripheral vascular resistance Increased blood pressure Mydriasis Increased tone of internal sphincter of bladder	Inhibits the release of: Norepinephrine Acetylcholine Insulin	Tachycardia Increased force of myocardial contraction Lipolysis Increases renin production – causes vasoconstriction.	Vasodilation Decreased peripheral vascular resistance Bronchodilation Glycogenolysis Increased secretion of glucagon Uterine smooth muscle relaxation

DIRECTLY ACTING ADRENERGIC AGONISTS:

Kinetics of endogenous norepinephrine:

- Norepinephrine is synthesized from dopamine. Dopamine is synthesized from the amino acid tyrosine. Tyrosine is transported from plasma into the adrenergic neuron, where the enzyme tyrosine hydroxylase converts it into DOPA (dihydroxyphenylalanine). The enzyme DOPA decarboxylase then converts this into dopamine.

- Dopamine is stored in synaptic vesicles, and norepinephrine is synthesized within the vesicles. The enzyme dopamine β-hydroxylase converts dopamine into norepinephrine.

- The mechanism of release is similar to acetylcholine. An action potential triggers calcium influx into the cell, which in turn causes the synaptic vesicle to fuse with the cell membrane and release its contents into the synaptic cleft.

- Norepinephrine interacts with postsynaptic receptors, and initiates a cascade of events through second messengers. Interaction with the presynaptic receptors regulates further release of norepinephrine.

- Final fate of norepinephrine:

  o It may be absorbed into systemic circulation.

o It may be taken back into the neuron. Here it can either be stored in the synaptic vesicle again, or undergo degradation through the enzyme monoamine oxidase.
o It may be degraded in the synaptic space itself by the enzyme catechol o-methyltransferase.

EPINEPHRINE:

This is a naturally occurring hormone that is formed by methylation of norepinephrine in the adrenal medulla. Epinephrine acts at both α and β receptors. At low doses, β effects predominate, while at higher doses, α effects predominate.

Clinical effects:
- CVS: Increases myocardial contractility. It stimulates renin production. There is vasoconstriction of the skin, mucous membranes, and visceral blood vessels, as well as of the kidney, but vasodilation of vessels leading to liver and skeletal muscles. Overall, there is an increase in systolic blood pressure but mild drop in the diastolic pressure.
- Respiratory: Causes powerful bronchodilation.
- Prevents release of histamine from mast cells.
- Hyperglycemia occurs due to glycogenolysis, increased secretion of glucagon, and decreased secretion of insulin.
- Increase in plasma levels of free fatty acids and glycerol due to lipolysis.

Pharmacokinetics:
- This is usually given parenterally, intramuscularly, or, in acute emergencies, intravenously. It may also be given through the subcutaneous route or by inhalation. Onset of action is rapid, followed by a brief duration of action. It is rapidly metabolized by MAO and COMT, and metabolites are excreted in urine.

Adverse effects:
- CNS effects: Headache, tension, fear, anxiety, tremors
- Cardiac arrhythmias
- Pulmonary edema

Indications:
- Because of its powerful effects, epinephrine is the drug of choice for several medical emergencies, which include:
- Life-threatening bronchospasm that occurs in asthma and anaphylaxis
- Cardiac arrest: To restore normal rhythm

- Local anesthetic supplementation: It is combined with local anesthetic drugs used for injection. This gives the following benefits:
  o Increases duration of action of local anesthetics by preventing plasma clearance of the drug.
  o Decreases systemic toxicity of local anesthetics.
  o Provides bloodless field for surgery.

NOREPINEPHRINE:

When administered as an external agent, norepinephrine influences only α receptors.

Clinical effects:

- CVS: Intense vasoconstriction and increase in peripheral vascular resistance cause rise in both systolic and diastolic blood pressure. The high blood pressure can stimulate baroreceptors, which may then stimulate the vagus nerve to lower the blood pressure.

Pharmacokinetics:

- It is usually given intravenously. Like adrenaline, it is rapidly metabolized by MAO and COMT and the metabolites are excreted in urine.

Adverse effects:

- Apart from the side effects produced by adrenaline, it may also cause sloughing or necrosis of the tissue into which it is injected.

Indications:

- Treatment of shock – helps increase peripheral vascular resistance.

DOPAMINE:

Like epinephrine, dopamine stimulates β receptors at low doses and α receptors at high doses. In addition, it also stimulates peripheral dopaminergic receptors.

Clinical effects:

- CVS: It has positive inotropic and chronotropic effects.
- By acting through dopaminergic receptors, it increases renal, splanchnic, and visceral blood flow.

Indications:

- Cardiogenic and septic shock: It increases systemic circulation without compromising visceral and renal blood flow.

Adverse effects:

- Nausea

- Hypertension and arrhythmias

DOBUTAMINE:

- This is a synthetic drug that acts exclusively on β1 receptors.
- It increases myocardial rate and contractility. It has no effect on vasculature.
- It is useful in acute heart failure, and to improve cardiac output after surgery.
- It can increase conduction rate, and must therefore not be used in atrial fibrillation.

OXYMETAZOLINE:

- This stimulates α1 and α2 receptors.
- This drug is largely used topically. It provides vasoconstriction of tissues, and can relieve congestion. However, long-term use can cause rebound congestion and dependence.
- In the form of nasal sprays, it is used as a decongestant. In the form of ophthalmic drops, it is used to decrease redness in the eyes.
- The drug may be absorbed into systemic circulation, and it can cause nervousness, headaches, and insomnia.

PHENYLEPHRINE:

- This drug selectively stimulates α1 receptors and raises both systolic and diastolic blood pressures. It may induce reflex bradycardia.
- It is used for treatment of hypotension, especially when it presents with tachycardia.
- Taken orally or topically in the form of a spray, it is used as a nasal decongestant.

ISOPROTERENOL:

- This drug non selectively stimulates β1 and β2 receptors. It does not have much effect on α receptors.
- Its actions on the heart and vasculature are similar to epinephrine. It raises systolic blood pressure and causes a slight drop in diastolic blood pressure. It is also a potent bronchodilator.
- Its therapeutic use is restricted to treatment of atrioventricular block.

CLONIDINE:

- Clonidine is a specific α2 agonist. It therefore is mainly involved in inhibition of neurotransmitters such as norepinephrine, acetylcholine, and the hormone insulin.

- This drug is used in the management of hypertension. However, abrupt cessation of the drug can cause rebound hypertension.
- This drug has also been used to manage withdrawal from habit-forming substances, including tobacco, opiates, and benzodiazepines.
- Adverse effects include lethargy, constipation, sedation, and xerostomia.

ALBUTEROL AND TERBUTALINE:

- These are β2 agonists, and their main effect is bronchodilation.
- They have a short duration of action and are primarily used via the inhalational route for managing acute asthma attacks.
- Terbutaline has also been used as a uterine relaxant. However, systemic administration may stimulate β1 receptors, and may cause arrhythmias and tachycardia.
- Side effects include tremors, restlessness, apprehension, and anxiety.

SALMETEROL AND FORMOTEROL:

- These are also β2 agonists, but they have a longer duration of action.
- They are used as maintenance therapy in asthma, in combination with corticosteroids.

INDIRECTLY ACTING ADRENERGIC AGONISTS:

These drugs potentiate the action of epinephrine and norepinephrine at their receptors. The main drugs in this category are the amphetamines.

Mechanism of action:

- These drugs stimulate the release of norepinephrine from the nerve membrane into the synapse. They also inhibit MAO, which in turn prevents degradation of norepinephrine.

Clinical effects:

- CNS: Stimulation of all areas of the brain leads to decreased sleepiness and fatigue, alertness, and decreased appetite.
- Sympathetic actions: These are similar to epinephrine and norepinephrine and include raised blood pressure and cardiac output.

Pharmacokinetics:

- The drug is fully absorbed through the oral route. It easily enters the CNS. Metabolism occurs in the liver and metabolites are excreted in urine.

Adverse effects:

- Dizziness, tremors, confusion, and panic
- Anorexia, nausea, vomiting, abdominal cramps, and diarrhea
- Hypertension, cardiac arrhythmias, circulatory collapse

Indications:

- Attention deficit hyperactivity disorder
- Narcolepsy

MIXED ACTION ADRENERGIC AGONISTS:

EPHEDRINE AND PSEUDOEPHEDRINE:

These drugs stimulate both α and β receptors. Moreover, they stimulate the release of norepinephrine from the nerve endings into the synapse.

Clinical effects:

- Increase in systolic and diastolic blood pressure.
- Bronchodilation
- CNS stimulation: Increases alertness, decreases sleep and fatigue.

Pharmacokinetics:

- These drugs are absorbed well orally. They can penetrate the blood-brain barrier and enter the brain. While ephedrine is not metabolized, pseudoephedrine undergoes partial metabolism in the liver. The drugs are eliminated in the urine.

Indications:

- Hypotension
- Pseudoephedrine is used as a decongestant.

ADRENERGIC ANTAGONISTS

These drugs bind either reversibly or irreversibly to the adrenergic receptors. They may be categorized as α blockers and β blockers.

α BLOCKERS:

These drugs cause a decrease in peripheral vascular resistance and hypotension. This in turn results in reflex tachycardia. Some common α blockers are described below:

PHENOXYBENZAMINE:

- This drug irreversibly blocks both α1 and α2 receptors. The actions of this drug can be reversed only after the body synthesizes new adrenoreceptors. This takes about 24 hours.
- It is primarily used for the medical management of pheochromocytoma (a tumor which secretes catecholamines). It is used both in inoperable cases, and prior to tumor removal to avoid hypertensive crises.
- It is also used to improve blood circulation in Raynaud's disease and frostbite.
- Adverse effects include nausea, vomiting, nasal stuffiness, and postural hypotension.

PHENTOLAMINE:

- When injected, this drug reversibly blocks both α1 and α2 receptors. The effect lasts for about four hours.
- It is contraindicated in patients with coronary artery disease, as it can induce arrhythmias and angina.
- Used in the treatment of hypertensive crisis, especially that induced by clonidine withdrawal and tyramine poisoning.
- It may also be used for the management of pheochromocytoma.

SELECTIVE α1 BLOCKERS:

- A group of drugs, including prazosin, terazosin, tamsulosin, and alfuzosin, selectively blocks only the α1 receptor.
- They decrease blood pressure and lower peripheral vascular resistance largely by acting on the smooth muscles of blood vessel walls. They do not affect cardiac output and renal blood flow.
- They also relax muscles of the prostate and bladder, and improve flow of urine.
- They are used as add-on drugs for the management of hypertension.
- They can cause nasal congestion, headache, drowsiness, and orthostatic hypotension.

YOHIMBINE:

- This is a selective α2 blocker.
- It is believed to be effective in the treatment of erectile dysfunction.
- It has the potential to worsen cardiovascular disease, renal dysfunction, and psychiatric disorders.

β BLOCKERS:

- β blockers may be either non-selective blockers (which block both β1 and β2), or they may be cardioselective blockers (block only β1).

NON-SELECTIVE β BLOCKERS:

Some drugs in this category include propranolol, nadolol, timolol, and carteolol.

Clinical effects:

- CVS: They have negative inotropic and chronotropic effects. The cardiac workload and oxygen consumption decreases, and there is bradycardia and lowering of blood pressure.
- Respiratory: They can cause bronchoconstriction and can exacerbate dyspnea in patients with lung disease.
- Endocrine: These drugs decrease glycogenolysis and secretion of glucagon, thereby lowering blood glucose levels. Caution must be used when prescribing these drugs to diabetic patients on insulin.

Pharmacokinetics:

- These drugs are usually taken orally. Propranolol usually undergoes extensive first-pass metabolism, with only 25% of the drug available to exert clinical effects. Metabolism occurs in the liver and metabolites are excreted in urine.

Adverse effects:

- Can cause significant bronchoconstriction.
- Abrupt cessation can lead to cardiac arrhythmias.
- May induce hypoglycemia.
- CNS effects: Depression, lethargy, dizziness, and visual disturbances.

Indications:

- Prevention of angina and myocardial infarction.
- Primary management of patients with hypertension.
- Supraventricular cardiac arrhythmias.
- Migraine: Propranolol can penetrate the CNS and is most useful for this purpose.
- Hyperthyroidism: They reduce sympathetic stimulation, and are protective against arrhythmias.
- Glaucoma: Nadolol and timolol are more potent, and therefore, are quite effective topically in diminishing intraocular pressure. These drugs also reduce the secretion of aqueous humor in the eye.

SELECTIVE β1 ANTAGONIST:

These drugs are also called cardioselective drugs, because they affect primarily the heart. Some drugs in this category include atenolol, acebutolol, esmolol, bisoprolol, and metoprolol.

Clinical effects:

- They have negative inotropic and chronotropic effects, and they lower blood pressure.
- They do not have any effect on pulmonary function, glucose metabolism, or peripheral vascular resistance.

Indications:

- Hypertensive patients who have impaired pulmonary function.
- Primary treatment for stable angina.
- Chronic heart failure

COMBINED α AND β ANTAGONISTS:

- Labetalol and carvedilol are drugs that block both α and β adrenergic receptors.
- They have the clinical effect of lowering blood pressure, while at the same time producing peripheral vasodilation.
- Labetalol is useful in pregnancy hypertension.
- Carvedilol is more useful in chronic heart failure, as it prevents vessel wall thickening in addition to reducing sympathetic stimulation of the heart.
- Adverse effects include dizziness and orthostatic hypotension

EXERCISES

1. Which of the following drugs cannot be used in an acute asthma attack?
   a. Albuterol
   b. Formoterol
   c. Adrenaline
   d. Terbutaline

2. Which of the following drugs effectively restores rhythm after cardiac arrest?
   a. Isoproterenol
   b. Adrenaline
   c. Dopamine
   d. Noradrenaline

3. Which of the following drugs increases cardiac output without compromising renal blood flow?
   a. Isoproterenol
   b. Adrenaline
   c. Dopamine
   d. Noradrenaline

4. Which of the following drugs is effective as a nasal spray decongestant?
   a. Phenylephrine
   b. Oxymetazoline
   c. Pseudoephedrine
   d. Adrenaline

5. Which of the following drugs acts at the adrenergic receptors, and also stimulates the release of neurotransmitters?
   a. Phenylephrine
   b. Isoproterenol
   c. Oxymetazoline
   d. Ephedrine

6. What is the bioavailability of oral propranolol?
   a. 10%
   b. 25%
   c. 50%
   d. 75%

7. Which of the following drugs inhibits both α and β adrenergic receptors?
   a. Propranolol
   b. Atenolol
   c. Labetalol
   d. Esmolol

8. Which of the following drugs is useful for managing hypertension in pregnancy?
   a. Esmolol
   b. Labetalol
   c. Atenolol
   d. Isoproterenol

9. Which of the following drugs used for management of hypertension is actually an adrenergic agonist?
   a. Propranolol
   b. Clonidine
   c. Atenolol
   d. Labetalol

10. Which of the following drugs are used in the management of attention deficit hyperactivity disorder?
    a. Amphetamine
    b. Clonidine
    c. Dopamine
    d. Atropine

UNIT IV : PERIPHERAL NERVOUS SYSTEM

CHAPTER 1

Local Anesthetics

Local anesthetics are a group of drugs which, when they are applied to a specific part of the body, cause reversible loss of sensation in that body part. They are classically used to 'numb' body parts when minor interventions are required. They may be injected, or applied topically as a spray or gel. Based on their chemical structure, local anesthetics are categorized into ester-linked drugs and amide-linked drugs (Table 1).

Table 1. Classification of local anesthetics

ESTER-LINKED LOCAL ANESTHETICS	AMIDE-LINKED LOCAL ANESTHETICS
Procaine	Lidocaine
Chloroprocaine	Prilocaine
Tetracaine	Mepivacaine
Benzocaine	Bupivacaine
	Articaine

MECHANISM OF ACTION:

Local anesthetics interfere with depolarization of the nerve. These drugs bind to receptors located on the inner side of transmembrane sodium channels. This blocks sodium ions from entering into the neuronal cell, which is essential for depolarization to take place. This in turn results in failure of the nerve to generate an action potential and conduct a nerve impulse.

PROPERTIES OF LOCAL ANESTHETICS THAT AFFECT THEIR ACTION:

- **pKa** : The local anesthetic molecule exists in two forms – the base form and ionized form. While the base form alone can penetrate to the interior of the cell, the ionized form binds to the receptor on the sodium channel. An equilibrium usually exists between the two forms. In general, drugs with lower pKa have a faster onset of action.

- **Lipid solubility** : If the base form is more lipid soluble, it can easily penetrate the nerve membrane. This increases drug potency.

- **Protein binding** : The greater the protein binding, the longer the time that the ionized form remains attached to the receptor site. This increases the duration of action of the anesthetic drug.

- **Non-nervous tissue distribution, and vasodilation** : Both these factors divert the local anesthetic away from the site of action, decreasing the duration of action.

- Based on their potency and duration of action, local anesthetics may be classified as follows:

  o Low potency and short duration of action: Procaine, Chloroprocaine
  o Intermediate potency and duration: Lignocaine, Prilocaine
  o High potency and long duration: Tetracaine, Bupivacaine, Ropivacaine

CLINICAL EFFECTS:

Local effects:
- Local anesthetics block nerve impulse transmission in sensory, somatic, and autonomic nerves.
- They also reduce the release of acetylcholine at the neuromuscular junction, which can cause temporary muscle paralysis.
- Sensations are blocked in the following order: pain, temperature, touch, deep pressure.

Systemic effects:
- **CNS**: Local anesthetics initially stimulate the CNS, and then depress it. Stimulation occurs due to inhibition of inhibitory neurons. Stimulation is most powerful with cocaine, and can manifest as excitement, euphoria, restlessness, mental confusion, tremors, twitching, and convulsions. With other drugs like lignocaine, there is circumoral numbness, abnormal tongue sensation, blurred vision, and tinnitus. CNS depression manifests as lethargy, dysphoria, drowsiness, and loss of consciousness.
- **CVS**: Local anesthetics do not have cardiac effects at normal doses. At high doses, they decrease myocardial conduction and contractility. Some drugs like lignocaine shorten the refractory period, and have an antiarrhythmic effect. On the other hand, bupivacaine can cause ventricular tachycardia and fibrillation.

- **Blood vessels**: Local anesthetics cause vasodilation. At low doses, this is due to the effect of blocking sympathetic conduction. At higher doses, the drug directly causes relaxation of the smooth muscles of the vessel wall.

Pharmacokinetics:

Local anesthetics are either applied or injected topically at the site of action. Some drugs are absorbed systemically through the vascularity of that region, and are widely distributed.

Amide-linked local anesthetics bind to α1 glycoproteins in plasma. They are metabolized in the liver by dealkylation and hydrolysis. Ester-linked local anesthetics are degraded in the plasma itself by the enzyme pseudocholinesterase.

Adverse Effects:

Usually adverse effects are only noted when a large volume of the drug is absorbed systemically. This may occur with inadvertent injections of the anesthetic into a blood vessel. These include:

- Dizziness, confusion, visual and auditory disturbances, twitching, tremors and convulsions. At toxic doses, respiratory arrest can occur.
- Bradycardia, hypotension, arrhythmias
- Ester-linked anesthetics may cause hypersensitivity reactions.

Indications:

It is used to provide 'numbness' during interventional procedures. There are several different techniques of producing local anesthesia. These are summarized in Table 2.

Table 2. Techniques of local anesthesia administration

TECHNIQUE	METHOD	USES
Surface anesthesia	The local anesthetic, in the form of creams, gels, or sprays, is directly applied to the surface. It also includes eye/ear drops.	Mucosal ulcers and abrasions, pain relief.
Infiltration	The anesthetic solution is deposited subcutaneously directly into the area of intervention. This blocks free nerve endings.	Small incisions, suturing lacerations, dental procedures.

105

Field block	This is a subcutaneous injection, which blocks all the nerves entering a particular field.	Larger incisions and suturing procedures
Nerve block	The anesthetic solution is injected near the main trunk of a nerve or one of its specific branches.	Dental and ophthalmic procedures
Spinal anesthesia	The anesthetic is injected directly into the subarachnoid space. It causes anesthesia and paralysis of the lower abdomen and limbs.	Surgical procedures on the lower abdomen, pelvis and lower limbs.
Epidural anesthesia	The anesthetic is injected into the epidural space. It acts similar to spinal anesthesia, but requires greater volumes of drug, and is more technically demanding.	Obstetric purposes Postoperative pain relief

CONTRAINDICATIONS:

- Mepivacaine can cause toxicity to the newborn child. It must be avoided for obstetrics procedures.
- **Liver dysfunction**: Amide local anesthetics must be avoided.

EXERCISES

1. Which of the following drugs is not an amide local anesthetic?
   a. Lignocaine
   b. Articaine
   c. Procaine
   d. Mepivacaine

2. Which of the following ion channels is blocked by local anesthetics?
   a. Sodium
   b. Calcium
   c. Magnesium
   d. Chloride

3. Which of the following is true of the local anesthetic tetracaine?
   a. Low potency
   b. Intermediate potency
   c. High potency
   d. Intermediate duration of action

4. Which of the following properties increases the potency of the local anesthetic drug?
   a. Lipid solubility
   b. Water solubility
   c. Low pKa
   d. High pKa

5. Which of the following is dependent on the pKa of the local anesthetic?
   a. Onset of action
   b. Duration of action
   c. Potency
   d. Adverse effect profile

6. Which of the following local anesthetics has an antiarrhythmic effect?
   a. Articaine
   b. Lignocaine
   c. Mepivacaine
   d. Bupivacaine

7. Where does metabolism of ester linked local anesthetics take place?
   a. Liver
   b. Skeletal muscle
   c. Kidney
   d. Plasma

8. Which of the following anesthetic techniques targets free nerve endings?
   a. Infiltration
   b. Nerve block
   c. Spinal block
   d. Epidural block

9. Which of the following anesthetic techniques is suitable for obstetric procedures?
   a. Infiltration
   b. Nerve block
   c. Spinal block
   d. Epidural block

10. Which of the following local anesthetics is contraindicated in pregnant women?
    a. Articaine
    b. Lignocaine
    c. Mepivacaine
    d. Bupivacaine

CHAPTER 2

Skeletal Muscle Relaxants

These are drugs that inhibit activity at the neuromuscular junction. They can reduce muscular tone, and can cause reversible paralysis. Depending on their site of action, they may be classified as peripherally acting muscle relaxants, or centrally acting muscle relaxants.

PERIPHERALLY ACTING MUSCLE RELAXANTS

Peripherally acting muscle relaxants are of two types – neuromuscular blocking agents and directly acting agents.

NEUROMUSCULAR BLOCKING AGENTS

These drugs act at the nicotinic receptors of the neuromuscular junction. Based on their mechanism of action, they are further classified as non-depolarizing, or depolarizing blockers.

NON-DEPOLARIZING BLOCKERS

These drugs are competitive antagonists for acetylcholine. At low doses, they bind to nicotinic receptors instead of acetylcholine, but do not stimulate the receptor. Therefore, muscle contraction does not occur. At high doses, they also block the ion channels. While low doses can be reversed by cholinesterases, high doses make reversal difficult.

Clinical actions:
- The main clinical action is paralysis of muscles.
- Muscle paralysis occurs in a centrifugal manner, starting with the muscles of the eye and face, followed by fingers and toes. After that, muscles of the limbs are affected, and finally, paralysis of the neck and trunk muscles occurs.

109

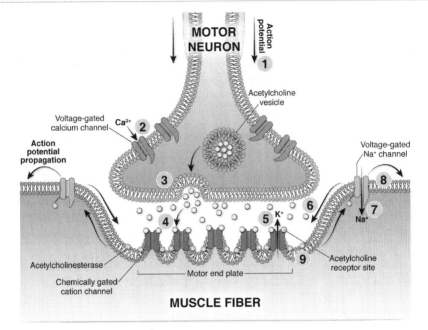

Neuromuscular Junction

1. An action potential is propagated down the motor neuron.

2. The action potential triggers the opening of voltage-gated calcium channels, and calcium enters the terminal button of the motor neuron.

3. Calcium triggers the release of acetylcholine by exocytosis.

4. Acetylcholine diffuses across the space between the neuron and muscle and binds with receptors on the muscle cell's motor end plate.

5. The binding opens cation channels, and a relatively large amount of Na⁺ moves into the muscle cell compared to a smaller movement of K⁺ outward.

6. This causes an end-plate potential.

7. The end-plate potential opens voltage-gated Na⁺ channels.

8. Na⁺ entry reduces the potential to threshold; action potential is propagated.

9. Acetylcholine is destroyed by acetylcholinesterase, ending muscle cell's response.

Figure 7 Skeletal muscle relaxants act on receptors of the neuromuscular junction, the synapse between a motor neuron and muscle fiber. Under typical circumstances, the motor neuron transmits a signal to the muscle fiber, causing muscle contraction. Skeletal muscle relaxants inhibit activity at the neuromuscular junction, ultimately reducing muscular tone and causing reversible paralysis.

Pharmacokinetics:

These drugs are not effective when taken orally. They are usually administered intravenously, and sometimes, intramuscularly. They are selectively distributed to the muscles and do not penetrate membranes, including the blood brain barrier. They are usually not metabolized, and are excreted unchanged in the urine. Based on their duration of action, these drugs are classified as:

- Long acting: Pancuronium, pipercuronium, doxacurium
- Intermediate acting: Vecuronium, rocuronium, atracurium
- Short acting: Mivacurium

Adverse effects:

- Postoperative muscle pain
- Hypokalemia
- Increased intraocular and intragastric pressure

Indications:

- Non-depolarizing blockers are commonly used during general anesthesia to maintain a state of muscle relaxation that is conducive to intubation and surgery.

DEPOLARIZING BLOCKERS:

These agents are agonists for acetylcholine. They work similar to acetylcholine, and cause depolarization of the motor end plate. However, while acetylcholine degrades rapidly, these agents are resistant to degradation. The continuous depolarization prevents the transmission of further nerve impulses, by closing off the sodium channel. The main depolarizing blocker in use today is succinylcholine.

Clinical actions:

- These are similar to depolarizing agents. There might be mild fasciculations or twitching of the muscles before paralysis sets in.

Pharmacokinetics:

- Succinylcholine is usually administered intravenously. After it acts at the neuromuscular junction, it rapidly redistributes, and is hydrolyzed in plasma by the enzyme pseudocholinesterase. The duration of action lasts only up to five minutes.

Adverse effects:

- Succinylcholine has the potential to induce malignant hyperthermia

- Apnea: Certain susceptible patients may not be able to metabolize succinylcholine. This occurs in patients who have a genetically altered form of the enzyme pseudocholinesterase. Patients who have electrolyte disturbances, or those receiving digoxin may also be susceptible to apnea.
- Hyperkalemia.

Indications:
- Used along with rapid endotracheal intubation, during induction of general anesthesia.

DIRECTLY ACTING MUSCLE RELAXANTS

Rather than acting at the neuromuscular junction, these drugs act on the muscles themselves. The important drug in this category is dantrolene sodium.

Dantrolene:
- This drug blocks the calcium channels present on the sarcoplasmic reticulum of skeletal muscles. This decreases intracellular calcium available for excitation-contraction coupling, and inhibits muscle contraction.
- It may be given either orally or intravenously. It is well absorbed from the GIT, and can penetrate the brain. It is metabolized in the liver and excreted by the kidney. The half life is 8 to 12 hours.
- Adverse effects include sedation, weakness, muscle weakness and diarrhea.
- Indications:
  o Oral dantrolene: Hemiplegia, paraplegia, cerebral palsy and multiple sclerosis to reduce spasticity.
  o Intravenous dantrolene: drug of choice for malignant hyperthermia.

CENTRALLY ACTING MUSCLE RELAXANTS

These drugs act on the spinal and supraspinal polysynaptic pathways that are responsible for maintenance of muscle tone. They decrease muscle tone and cause some sedation, but do not affect the neuromuscular transmission and hence do not cause complete paralysis. Some commonly used skeletal muscle relaxants include:

Chlorzoxazone:
- It is used to relieve painful muscle spasms, and increase joint mobility.
- It undergoes glucuronide conjugation by the liver, and is excreted in urine.
- Side effects include: nausea, vomiting, light-headedness, headache, drowsiness.

Chlormezanone:

- Primarily used for muscle spasm, it has anti-anxiety and hypnotic actions as well.
- Side effects: Nausea, abdominal pain, fatigue, dizziness. At toxic doses, it can cause cerebral edema, liver and kidney damage.

Thiocolchicoside:

- Apart from being a muscle relaxant, it has anti-inflammatory and analgesic effects.
- It is administered orally, and bioavailability is 25%. It is metabolized in plasma, and excreted through urine and feces.
- Can induce seizures and is contraindicated in patients with epilepsy.

Tizanidine:

- It has a short duration of action, and is used to relieve muscle spasticity before specific activities.
- It is absorbed orally, with a bioavailability of 40%. It undergoes significant first pass metabolism, and is 30% bound to plasma proteins. It is metabolized in the liver and excreted in urine.
- Can increase the heart rate and blood pressure.
- Benzodiazepines and other drugs acting on the CNS: These include diazepam and baclofen, which have been described in Unit II.

EXERCISES

1. Which of the following drugs is not a non-depolarizing blocker?
   a. Pancuronium
   b. Vecuronium
   c. Succinylcholine
   d. Atracrium

2. What action do non-depolarizing blockers have on the nicotinic receptors?
   a. Agonist
   b. Antagonist
   c. Neither
   d. Both agonist and antagonist

3. Which of the following is a short acting non-depolarizing blocker?
   a. Atracurium
   b. Mivacurium
   c. Doxacurium
   d. Pancuronium

4. What is the preferred route of administration for peripheral muscle relaxants?
   a. Oral
   b. Intramuscular
   c. Intravenous
   d. Subcutaneous

5. What is the duration of action of succinylcholine?
   a. 2 minutes
   b. 5 minutes
   c. 8 minutes
   d. 10 minutes

6. What is the drug of choice to treat malignant hyperthermia?
   a. Quinine
   b. Dantolene
   c. Tizanidine
   d. Chlorzoxazone

7. What is the half-life of dantrolene sodium?
   a. 2 to 4 hours
   b. 4 to 8 hours
   c. 8 to 12 hours
   d. 12 to 16 hours

8. Which of the following drugs has analgesic properties?
   a. Chlorzoxazone
   b. Tizanidine
   c. Thiocolchicoside
   d. Chlormezanone

9. Which of the following drugs can cause anxiolysis and sedation?
   a. Chlorzoxazone
   b. Tizanidine
   c. Thiocolchicoside
   d. Chlormezanone

10. Which of the following drugs is contraindicated in seizure patients?
    a. Chlorzoxazone
    b. Tizanidine
    c. Thiocolchicoside
    d. Chlormezanone

UNIT V : DRUGS ACTING ON THE PARACRINE AND ENDOCRINE SYSTEM

---------------------- CHAPTER 1 ----------------------

Histamine and Antihistamines

The current unit deals with paracrine (autacoid) drugs and endocrine drugs. Paracrine, or autacoid compounds are those which act locally at the site where they are released. In contrast, endocrine compounds, or hormones, act at sites distant from where they are produced.

HISTAMINE

Histamine is a paracrine chemical messenger. It is found in mast cells and basophils, which are distributed in tissues all over the body. Tissues that contain high amounts of histamine include the skin, gastric mucosa, lungs, liver, and placenta. Histamine is also present outside of the mast cells, in regions such as the brain. While histamine is not used clinically, it is essential to understand the properties of this compound to understand the applications of antihistamine drugs.

Synthesis and storage:
- Synthesis occurs within mast cells, from the amino acid histidine. The reaction is catalyzed by the enzyme histidine decarboxylase. After synthesis, histamine is stored in granules within the mast cells.

Mechanism of action:
- Histamine is released from mast cells upon stimulation by toxins, micro-organisms, or trauma. Upon release, histamine exerts its effects through four classes of histamine receptors – H1, H2, H3, and H4. The clinical actions have been detailed only for three receptors, and only H1 and H2 have effective antagonists.

Table 1. Clinical effects mediated through different histamine receptors

	H1	H2	H3
CLINICAL EFFECTS MODULATED	Smooth muscle contraction Blood vessels: Vasoconstriction of larger vessels, due to its action on smooth muscles Vasodilation due to release of nitric oxide Stimulation of afferent nerve endings Stimulation of ganglionic cells Release of catecholamines from adrenal medulla Neurotransmitter in the brain	Gastric acid secretion Vasodilation Positive chronotropic and inotropic effect on the heart Uterine relaxation Neurotransmitter in the brain	Present at presynaptic region, inhibits further histamine release and causes sedation Inhibits acetylcholine release in intestines

ANTIHISTAMINES

Depending on the receptor at which drugs exert their clinical effects, antihistamines are broadly categorized as H1 antihistamines and H2 antihistamines.

H1 ANTIHISTAMINES

Mechanism of action:

- H1 antihistamines block the receptor-mediated response of histamine. These drugs are divided into two main categories:

- **First-generation drugs** : These drugs can penetrate the blood-brain barrier. They also tend to stimulate receptors other than the histamine receptors. Therefore, they may have more adverse effects. However, they are still used due to their low cost.

- **Second-generation drugs** : These drugs do not penetrate the blood-brain barrier easily. They specifically act only on the peripheral H1 receptors, and therefore have lesser adverse effects.

Clinical actions and indications:

- **Effect on inflammation and allergies** : H1 antihistamines prevent the interaction of antigens with IgE antibodies. Therefore, they are useful in preventing allergic conditions. These include urticaria, allergic rhinitis, and allergic conjunctivitis. In allergic conditions that involve massive release of histamine, such as anaphylaxis, epinephrine is preferred over H1 antihistamines.

- **CNS depression** : This is largely seen with the first-generation antihistamines. Some second-generation antihistamines, including cetirizine and levocetirizine, may be partially sedating. First-generation drugs such as diphenhydramine and doxylamine are often prescribed in the treatment of insomnia.

- **Motion sickness and nausea** : First-generation drugs that act on both the histamine and muscarinic M1 receptors are useful in treating motion sickness. The drugs of choice include promethazine, cyclizine, meclizine, diphenhydramine, and dimenhydrinate. Promethazine is also used to control nausea that occurs in pregnancy. Some antihistamines, such as cyproheptadine, may have an appetite stimulating effect.

- **Anticholinergic effects** : Some first-generation drugs, including diphenhydramine, dimenhydrinate, pheniramine, and promethazine act at muscarinic receptors and inhibit the effects of acetylcholine. This can cause dry mouth, blurred vision, and urinary retention.

Pharmacokinetics:

- These drugs are well absorbed from the oral route. They are widely distributed, and reach all tissues (except the brain in the case of second-generation agents). These drugs are mostly metabolized in the liver through the cytochrome P450 system. Cetirizine, levocetirizine, and fexofenadine do not undergo any metabolism. The former two are excreted unchanged in the urine, while the latter passes out unchanged through the feces. The drugs usually reach peak levels in plasma within one to two hours, and the half-life is usually 4 to 6 hours for first-generation drugs, and 12 to 24 hours for the second-generation drugs.

Adverse effects:

- **CNS effects** : First-generation drugs can cause sedation, fatigue, dizziness, tremors, and lack of coordination. These drugs must not be taken when people work jobs that require them to be alert. Second-generation drugs can cause headaches.

- **Antimuscarinic effects** : These drugs can cause dry mouth, blurred vision, urinary retention, and tachycardia.

- **Hypersensitivity reactions** : Contact dermatitis can occur on topical application.

H2 ANTIHISTAMINES

These drugs block the actions of histamine at the H2 receptor. Usually, they produce competitive antagonism. However, famotidine alone works through competitive-noncompetitive blockade of H2 receptors.

Clinical actions:

- The main effect of the H2 blockers is on the GIT. Histamine, along with acetylcholine and gastrin, stimulates gastric acid production. H2 blockers basically suppress gastric acid secretion. They decrease all phases of gastric acid secretion, including basal, gastric, neurogenic, and psychic phases.

Pharmacokinetics:

- Absorption occurs through the oral route. These drugs undergo first-pass metabolism, and so only have a bioavailability of 60% to 80%. They do not cross the blood-brain barrier, but they can cross the placenta, and are also secreted in breast milk. Some oxidative metabolism occurs, but the drug is largely excreted unchanged in bile and urine. The half-life is two to three hours.

Indications:

- **Peptic ulcers** : Gastric and duodenal ulcers can be treated with H2 blockers. However, ulcers induced by drugs like NSAIDS are resistant.

- **Stress ulcers** : H2 blockers are used to manage stress ulcers in hospitalized patients. Tolerance may develop on prolonged use.

- **Gastroesophageal reflux disease** : These are not the preferred choice, and have been replaced with antacids and proton pump inhibitors.

Adverse effects:

- **CNS** : Hallucinations and confusion observed basically in elderly patients or if the drug is given intravenously.

- Headache, dizziness, muscular pain, diarrhea

- **Endocrine effects** : Observed with cimetidine. These include gynecomastia, galactorrhea, and decreased sperm count.

- All H2 blockers except famotidine, interfere with the absorption of ketoconazole.

-------- EXERCISES --------

1. Which one of the following receptors is responsible for inhibition of further histamine release?
   a. H1
   b. H2
   c. H3
   d. H4

2. Which of the following receptors mediates uterine relaxation?
   a. H1
   b. H2
   c. H3
   d. H4

3. Which of the following antihistamine drugs does not cause sedation at all?
   a. Diphenhydramine
   b. Cetirizine
   c. Fexofenadine
   d. Chlorpheniramine

4. Which of the following is the most common adverse effect of second-generation H1 antihistamines?
   a. Nausea
   b. Weight gain
   c. Dizziness
   d. Headache

5. In addition to histamine receptors, which of the following receptors are stimulated by first-generation antihistamines?
   a. Adrenergic
   b. Muscarinic
   c. Dopaminergic
   d. Serotonin

6. Which of the following drugs is indicated to control nausea in pregnancy?
   a. Promethazine
   b. Dimenhydrinat
   c. Cyproheptadine
   d. Levocetirizine

7. Which of the following drugs does not undergo metabolism in the body, and is excreted through feces?
   a. Cetirizine
   b. Fexofenadine
   c. Meclizine
   d. Promethazine

8. Which of the following drugs is used as an appetite stimulant?
   a. Cyproheptadine
   b. Promethazine
   c. Pheniramine
   d. Meclizine

9. Which of the following is the primary indication for use of H2 antihistamines?
   a. Allergic rhinitis
   b. Sinusitis
   c. Peptic ulcer
   d. Asthma

10. What is the bioavailability of H2 antihistamines?
   a. 10 – 20%
   b. 20 – 40%
   c. 40 – 60%
   d. 60- 80%

Prostaglandins and Prostaglandin Inhibitors

Prostaglandins are autacoids that are produced by almost all the tissues in the body. Once they exert their actions at the site of synthesis, they are degraded rapidly.

SYNTHESIS OF PROSTAGLANDINS:

Prostaglandins are synthesized from arachidonic acid. This is a long-chain free fatty acid that is generally present as a component of cell membranes, and is cleaved from this region by the enzyme phospholipase A2. Arachidonic acid then enters one of two metabolic pathways:

- **Cyclooxygenase pathway** : The enzyme cyclooxygenase (COX) exists in two isoforms. COX-1 is responsible for prostaglandin production in normal health. COX-2 is responsible for prostaglandin production during inflammation, and its expression is influenced by the presence of inflammatory mediators, including tumor necrosis factor-α (TNF-α) and interleukin-1 (IL-1). The COX pathway produces three prostaglandins – PGD2, PGE2, PGF2, prostacyclin (PGI2), and thromboxane A2.

- **Lipoxygenase pathway** : The enzyme lipoxygenase acts on arachidonic acid to produce leukotrienes.

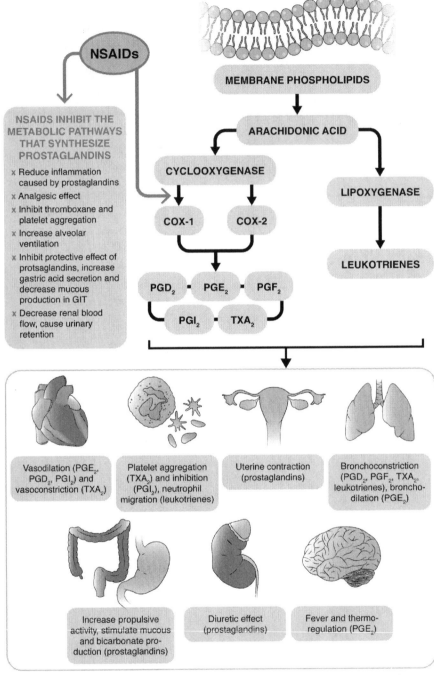

NSAIDs

MEMBRANE PHOSPHOLIPIDS

NSAIDS INHIBIT THE METABOLIC PATHWAYS THAT SYNTHESIZE PROSTAGLANDINS

x Reduce inflammation caused by prostaglandins
x Analgesic effect
x Inhibit thromboxane and platelet aggregation
x Increase alveolar ventilation
x Inhibit protective effect of protsaglandins, increase gastric acid secretion and decrease mucous production in GIT
x Decrease renal blood flow, cause urinary retention

ARACHIDONIC ACID

CYCLOOXYGENASE

LIPOXYGENASE

COX-1   **COX-2**

LEUKOTRIENES

PGD_2 - PGE_2 - PGF_2

PGI_2 - TXA_2

Vasodilation (PGE_2, PGD_2, PGI_2) and vasoconstriction (TXA_2)

Platelet aggregation (TXA_2) and inhibition (PGI_2), neutrophil migration (leukotrienes)

Uterine contraction (prostaglandins)

Bronchoconstriction (PGD_2, PGF_2, TXA_2, leukotrienes), bronchodilation (PGE_2)

Increase propulsive activity, stimulate mucous and bicarbonate production (prostaglandins)

Diuretic effect (prostaglandins)

Fever and thermoregulation (PGE_2)

Figure 8 Two metabolic pathways (COX and Lipoxygenase) produce prostaglandins that act on various systems in the body.

CLINICAL ACTIONS:

- **Cardiovascular system** : Most prostaglandins (PGE2, PGD2, and PGI2) cause vasodilation. Vasodilation results in a fall in blood pressure, which in turn causes an increase in cardiac output. PGF2α may cause vasoconstriction of larger vessels. Thromboxane A2 uniformly causes vasoconstriction. In the fetus, PGE2 production keeps the ductus arteriosus patent.

- **Injury and inflammation** : Thromboxanes can cause platelet aggregation, while prostacyclin tends to inhibit it. Both prostaglandins and leukotrienes are analgesic agents and they sensitize peripheral nerves to pain stimulus. They also modulate pain during inflammatory processes. Leukotrienes increase capillary permeability and cause neutrophil migration.

- **Smooth muscle contraction** : Prostaglandins cause uterine contraction, in gravid and non-gravid women. PGD2, PGF2α, and thromboxanes cause bronchoconstriction. However, PGE2 causes bronchodilation. Leukotrienes also cause bronchoconstriction.

- **GIT** : Prostaglandins increase propulsive activity of the GIT. They also stimulate the production of mucus and bicarbonate, and are protective against ulcers.

- **Renal system** : Prostaglandins have a diuretic effect. They increase the excretion of water, as well as sodium and potassium ions.

- **Nervous system** : Prostaglandins are pyrogenic and play a role in the development of fever. PGE2 is the main compound involved, and stimulates the hypothalamic thermoregulatory center to cause fever. Prostaglandins also modulate sympathetic transmission.

PROSTAGLANDIN ANALOGUES:

Synthetic forms of prostaglandins are used therapeutically for several purposes. A list of analogues, with their indications is summarized in Table 1.

Table 1. Prostaglandin analogues and their uses

DRUG	ANALOGUE OF	INDICATIONS
Alprostadil	PGE1	To maintain patent ductus arteriosus in infants with congenital heart conditions Treatment of erectile dysfunction
Lubiprostone	PGE1 derivative	Treatment of constipation: increases intestinal fluid secretion by stimulating chloride channels

Misoprostol	PGE1	Gastroprotective drug, given with NSAIDS in ulcer patients To induce labour in pregnant women
Bimatoprost Latanoprost Travoprost Tafluprost	PGF2α analogues	Treatment of open angle glaucoma Eyelash hypotrichosis
Epoprostenol Treprostinil	Prostacyclin	Treatment of pulmonary arterial hypertension

PROSTAGLANDIN INHIBITORS – NON-STEROIDAL ANTI-INFLAMMATORY DRUGS (NSAIDS)

NSAIDs are a group of drugs that exert clinical effects by inhibiting the metabolic pathways that synthesize prostaglandins. NSAIDs are classified according to their chemical structure and mechanism of action. This is summarized in Table 2.

Table 2. Classification of NSAIDS

DRUG CATEGORY	SUB-CATEGORY	DRUG NAMES
Non-selective COX inhibitors	Salicylates	Aspirin
	Propionic acid derivatives	Ibuprofen, Flurbiprofen, NaproxenMefenamic acid
	Fenemates	
	Enolic acid derivatives	Piroxicam, Tenoxicam
	Acetic acid derivatives	Indomethacin, Ketorolac
	Pyrazolone derivatives	Phenylbutazone, Oxyphenbutazone
Preferential COX-2 inhibitors		Nimesulide, diclofenac, aceclofenac, etodolac
Selective COX-2 inhibitors		Celecoxib, etoricoxib
Analgesic-antipyretics with poor anti-inflammatory action	Para-aminophenol derivative	Paracetamol
	Pyrazolone derivatives	Dipyrone, propyphenazone
	Benzoxazocine derivatives	Nefopam

Mechanism Of Action:

Most NSAIDs reversibly inhibit cyclooxygenase. Aspirin, however, alters the structure of the enzyme, and this action is irreversible.

Clinical Effects:

- **Anti-inflammatory agent** : NSAIDs reduce inflammation that is caused by prostaglandins. They are often used in inflammatory conditions like arthritis. While they do not slow the progression of the disease, they can improve symptoms.

- **Analgesic effect** : NSAIDs are the most common drugs used in pain management. Most analgesics are effective in the management of musculoskeletal pain. Some drugs, like ketorolac, are useful for severe acute pain.

- **Antipyretic effect** : NSAIDs reduce body temperature in patients with fever. They induce sweating and peripheral vasodilation, which rapidly dissipates heat.

- **CVS effects** : Low doses of aspirin inhibits thromboxane, which causes aggregation of platelets. It is therefore prescribed for patients who are at risk of developing ischemic events such as myocardial infarction or stroke. Aspirin is also used in acute myocardial infarction. It has been shown to reduce the size of the infarct and decrease mortality rates. Other non-selective NSAIDs can also inhibit platelet aggregation, but are not therapeutically useful. COX-2 inhibitors have no effect on platelets.

- **Respiratory effects** :
  o **Aclinical doses: Raised alveolar ventilation.**
  o **At high doses: Respiratory alkalosis compensated by the kidneys.**
  o **At toxic doses: Central respiratory paralysis.**

- **GIT effects** : They inhibit the protective effect of prostaglandins. They increase gastric acid secretion and decrease mucus production, thereby increasing the risk of developing ulcers.

- **Renal effects** : They decrease renal blood flow and can cause retention of sodium and water. This leads to urinary retention.

Pharmacokinetics:

Aspirin is degraded in various tissues of the body, including plasma, to form salicylate, which forms the active component. Salicylates are rapidly distributed throughout the body, and they cross the blood-brain barrier as well as the placenta. They are metabolized in the liver by conjugation reactions. They are excreted in the urine at the expense of uric acid, and can lead to accumulation of uric acid in the body.

Most of the other NSAIDs bind to plasma proteins and are metabolized in the liver. Excretion occurs through urine.

127

Table 3. Half-life and indications of various NSAIDs

DRUG	HALF-LIFE	INDICATIONS
Aspirin (as salicylate)	3 to 5 hours	Low dose – in ischemic diseases, acute rheumatic fever, and as an analgesic and antipyretic
Ibuprofen	2 hours	Mild to moderate postoperative pain
Naproxen	12 to 16 hours	Pain relief in patients with cardiovascular disease
Mefenemic acid	2 to 4 hours	Dysmenorrhoea. Pain in muscles, joints, soft tissues
Piroxicam	57 hours	Acute pain and musculoskeletal pain, long-term drug in inflammatory conditions
Ketorolac	5 to 7 hours	Acute postoperative pain, dental, musculoskeletal pain Reserve drug in inflammatory conditions
Indomethacin	2 to 5 hours	Fever refractory to other drugs Closure of patent ductus arteriosus
Nimesulide	2 to 5 hours	Pain of short duration – injuries, sinusitis
Diclofenac	2 hours, up to 6 hours in joints	Inflammatory pain – arthritis, bursitis, toothache, spondylitis
Etodolac	7 hours	Arthritis and musculoskeletal pain
Celecoxib	10 hours	Acute pain, rheumatoid arthritis, osteoarthritis
Etoricoxib	24 hours	Analgesic in patients with high risk of GI bleed
Paracetamol	2 to 3 hours	Antipyretic drug of choice. Analgesic in patients with gastric ulcers.

Adverse Effects:

- **Liver damage** : Paracetamol produces toxic metabolites, which can cause liver damage in high doses. Fulminant hepatic failure has also been reported with nimesulide.

- **Cardiovascular events** : The risk of events like myocardial infarction increases with COX-2 inhibitors.

- **Trigger for asthma** : Since NSAIDs suppress only prostaglandins, leukotrienes exert severe bronchoconstriction. This can trigger asthmatic attacks in susceptible patients.

- **Peptic ulcer** : The risk is higher with non-selective COX inhibitors.

- **Renal failure** : Patients with compromised renal function can develop renal failure.

- **Minor effects** : Headache and dizziness may occur with some drugs. Frontal headache is common with ketorolac. Some non-selective NSAIDs can cause hypersensitivity reactions like rashes.

Contraindications:

- Third trimester of pregnancy – can cause premature closure of ductus arteriosus
- Patients with gout, or those taking probenecid
- Patients at high risk of renal failure
- Patients with cardiovascular disease (COX-2 inhibitors are contraindicated)

EXERCISES

1. Which of the following fatty acids is a substrate for synthesis of prostaglandins?
   a. Linoleic acid
   b. Linolenic acid
   c. Arachidonic acid
   d. Eicosa-tetraenoic acid

2. Which of the following prostaglandins keeps the ductus arteriosus patent in the fetus?
   a. PGD2
   b. PGE2
   c. PGF2α
   d. PGI2

3. Which of the following drugs is a synthetic analog of PGF2α?
   a. Alprostadil
   b. Misoprostol
   c. Bimatoprost
   d. Epoprostenol

4. In which trimester of pregnancy is the use of NSAIDs contraindicated?
   a. First
   b. Second
   c. Third
   d. Throughout pregnancy

5. Which of the following NSAIDs is preferred for patients with cardiovascular disease?
   a. Ibuprofen
   b. Naproxen
   c. Diclofenac
   d. Etodolac

e. Which of the following NSAIDs has been associated with a high risk of cardiovascular events?

f. Aspirin

g. Indomethacin

h. Celecoxib

i. Ketorolac

6. Which of the following NSAIDs is used as a prophylaxis for ischemic events?

a. Aspirin

b. Indomethacin

c. Sulindac

d. Propyphenazone

7. Which of the following drugs causes frontal headache?

a. Diclofenac

b. Ketorolac

c. Piroxicam

d. Etoricoxib

8. What is the half-life of celecoxib?

a. 5 hours

b. 7 hours

c. 10 hours

d. 12 hours

9. Which NSAID is indicated for patients with pain due to dysmenorrhea?

a. Piroxicam

b. Indomethacin

c. Mefenamic acid

d. Aspirin

CHAPTER 3

Drugs Acting on the Hypothalamus and Pituitary Gland

This chapter deals with the hormones secreted by the hypothalamus and the pituitary gland. These areas secrete hormones which influence the production of hormones by the other endocrine glands. The hypothalamus secretes regulatory hormones, which are transmitted to the anterior pituitary via the hypothalamo-hypophyseal portal system. These hormones regulate secretion of hormones from the pituitary.

ANTERIOR PITUITARY HORMONES: ADRENOCORTICOTROPIC HORMONE (ACTH)

The hypothalamus secretes corticotropin releasing hormone (CRH), which acts on the anterior pituitary to secrete ACTH, also known as corticotropin.

Physiological function:

ACTH acts on receptors present on the surface of the adrenal cortex. By activating G-protein-coupled receptors, it stimulates the release of corticosteroids (Cortisol) and adrenergic hormones.

Cortisol has a negative feedback relationship with CRH and ACTH. If cortisol levels are high, they suppress CRH and ACTH release, which in turn suppresses cortisol secretion.

Therapeutic indications:
- Synthetic ACTH (cosyntropin) is used to diagnose adrenal insufficiency.
- It is also used in treating West Syndrome, a disease of infants that causes spasms.

GROWTH HORMONE (GH)

Somatotropin, also known as growth hormone, is produced by the anterior pituitary when it is stimulated by somatotropin-releasing-hormone produced by the hypothalamus. Another hypothalamic hormone, calles somatostatin, inhibits the secretion of this hormone.

Physiological effects:

Somatotropin has the following metabolic effects on tissue cells.

- It causes hyperplasia of tissues, and increases protoplasm production in cells.
- There is increased uptake of amino acids and protein synthesis.
- There is increased fat utilization and a tendency to spare carbohydrates.
- Increased gluconeogenesis and glycogenolysis.
- The above effects result in overall growth of bones as well as soft tissues.

Therapeutic indications:

Synthetic growth hormone is indicated in:

- GH deficiency and failure to grow
- AIDS wasting syndrome
- To improve athletic performance and enhance lean muscle mass.

SOMATOSTATIN

- This is an inhibitor of growth hormone. It is available in the synthetic form as octreotide and lanreotide.
- It is used for the management of acromegaly and bleeding esophageal varices.
- Adverse effects include nausea, diarrhea, steatorrhea, flatulence, and abdominal pain.

THYROID STIMULATING HORMONE (TSH)

Thyrotropin or TSH is released by the anterior pituitary, upon stimulation from the thyrotropin-releasing-hormone produced by the hypothalamus. It stimulates the thyroid gland to produce its hormones, triiodothyronine and thyroxine by the following mechanisms:

- Induces hypertrophy and hyperplasia of the thyroid cells.
- Improves blood supply to the thyroid gland.
- Increases trapping of iodine into the thyroid cells, and incorporation of iodine into the thyroid hormones.
- As such, it has no therapeutic application. It may sometimes be used for diagnosis, to differentiate primary hypothyroidism from hypothyroidism due to thyroid dysfunction.

GONADOTROPINS

The gonadotropin-releasing-hormone stimulates the release of gonadotropins from the anterior pituitary. The gonadotropins include follicle stimulating hormone (FSH) and luteinizing hormone (LH).

Physiological functions:

- In the ovaries, FSH induces follicular growth and development of the ovum. It also stimulates secretion of estrogen.

- In males, FSH supports spermatogenesis and development of the seminiferous tubules.

- LH supports ovulation and luteinization of the follicle. It maintains the integrity of the corpus luteum. It is also responsible for the secretion of progesterone.

- In males, the equivalent of LH is the interstitial cell stimulating hormone (ICSH). It is responsible for the secretion of testosterone.

Therapeutic indications:

- GnRH is available as synthetic analogs – leuprolide, goserelin, and histelin. They are used for suppression of gonadal hormones in conditions like prostate cancer, endometriosis, and precocious puberty.

- Gonadotropins are used for treatment of amenorrhea and infertility.

- **Hypogonadism and undescended testes** : Gonadotropins may induce androgens which can stimulate sexual maturation.

Adverse effects:

- GnRH analogs may cause decreased libido, hot flushes, sweating, gynecomastia, and ovarian cysts.

PROLACTIN

Prolactin has a negative feedback with GnRH. When high levels of prolactin are present, GnRH secretion is suppressed, and vice-versa.

Physiological function:

- During pregnancy, it stimulates the production of ductal and acinar cells in the breast. Within these cells, it stimulates the production of lactose and milk proteins.

- After delivery, it stimulates milk production. Prolactin is responsible for amenorrhoea during the lactation period. It can inhibit ovulation and fertility during this period.

Inhibitors of prolactin

- Bromocriptine and cabergoline are basically dopamine (D2) agonists. They bind to dopamine receptors on the pituitary and inhibit the release of prolactin.
- Bromocriptine is short acting and has a half-life of three to five hours. However, cabergoline has a half-life of almost 60 hours.
- These drugs are indicated in hyperprolactinemia due to prolactin secreting tumors. They are also used in acromegaly, and to some extent, in management of Parkinsonism.
- Adverse effects include nausea, vomiting, hypotension. and constipation.

POSTERIOR PITUITARY HORMONES

Oxytocin

- This hormone stimulates uterine contraction and is used in obstetrics to induce labor.
- Adverse effects include water retention, hypertension, and uterine rupture.

Vasopressin

- Also known as antidiuretic hormone, it plays a key role in urinary retention.
- It increases reabsorption of water in the collecting tubules of the kidney.
- It is mainly used to treat diabetes insipidus. It is used to manage bleeding from esophageal varices.
- Adverse effects include hyponatremia and water intoxication, abdominal pain and tremors. It causes vasoconstriction and may increase blood pressure. An analog of vasopressin, called desmopressin, does not cause vasoconstriction and is preferred for diabetes insipidus.

EXERCISES

1. Which of the following hormones is released by the hypothalamus?
   a. Adrenocorticotropihormone
   b. Corticotropin releasing hormone
   c. Cosyntropin
   d. Cortisol

2. Which of the following drugs is used in the management of acromegaly?
   a. Octreotide
   b. Cabergoline
   c. Leuprolide
   d. Desmopressin

3. Which of the following hormones maintains the integrity of the corpus luteum?
   a. Follicle stimulating hormone
   b. Luteinizing hormone
   c. Interstitial cell stimulating hormone
   d. Prolactin

4. Which of the following hormones is absent in men?
   a. Follicle stimulating hormone
   b. Luteinizing hormone
   c. Interstitial cell stimulating hormone
   d. Prolactin

5. Which of the following receptors, on activation, inhibits prolactin secretion?
   a. Adrenergic
   b. Dopaminergic
   c. Serotonin
   d. Muscarinic

6. Which of the following drugs is used to induce labour?
   a. Goserelin
   b. Bromocriptine
   c. Prolactin
   d. Oxytocin

7. Which of the following hormones is preferred for the treatment of diabetes insipidus?
   a. Prolactin
   b. Oxytocin
   c. Vasopressin
   d. Desmopressin

8. Which of the following drugs are used in the treatment of bleeding esophageal varices?
   a. Octreotide
   b. Vasopressin
   c. Lanreotide
   d. All of the above

9. What is the half-life of cabergoline?
   a. 20 hours
   b. 40 hours
   c. 60 hours
   d. 80 hours

10. Which of the following is not an adverse effect of vasopressin?
    a. Hyponatremia
    b. Dehydration
    c. Tremors
    d. Abdominal pain

CHAPTER 4

Thyroid Hormone and Inhibitors

The thyroid hormones, secreted by the thyroid gland, regulate basic metabolic processes throughout the body. The two major thyroid hormones are tri-iodothyronine (T3) and thyroxine (T4).

SYNTHESIS AND KINETICS:

The synthesis of these hormones involves the following steps:

- Dietary iodine is taken up into the thyroid cell through the Na^+ I symporter. Within the cell, it undergoes oxidation.
- Thyroglobulin is another protein that is synthesized within the cell.
- Iodine combines with the tyrosine residue of thyroglobulin to form monoiodothyronine and di-iodothyronine.
- The iodinated tyrosine residues then couple together to form T3 and T4. These hormones are stored in the thyroid follicles until they are released into circulation.
- In circulation, the hormones bind to thyroxine binding protein, and dissociate from it prior to entering the cell. Once within the cell, T4 is converted into T3. T3 exerts its action on the nucleus, and results in protein synthesis.
- T3 and T4 exert a negative feedback on TSH and TRH.
- Synthetic hormones are well absorbed after oral administration. They are metabolized by deiodination, and by conjugation with glucuronides and sulfates. Excretion occurs through the bile.

PHYSIOLOGICAL FUNCTIONS OF T3 AND T4:

- **Normal growth and development** : T3 and T4 are essential for normal growth of the body.
- **Metabolism** : These hormones enhance lipolysis and increase plasma free fatty acid levels. They also stimulate glycogenolysis and gluconeogenesis, leading to hyperglycemia. While they enhance synthesis of certain proteins, they also degrade

proteins to be used as a source of energy. Overall, they stimulate metabolism and increase the basal metabolic rate.

- **CVS** : They increase the heart rate, contractility, and cardiac output. Hyperthyroid patients may develop tachycardia, along with atrial fibrillation and congestive heart failure. Hypothyroid patients develop bradycardia. Hypothyroid patients may also develop anemia.

- **CNS** : Thyroid hormones boost mental function. Hypothyroid patients are sluggish and have impaired mental faculties. Hyperthyroid patients tend to be tense, anxious, and may develop tremors.

- **Skeletal muscle** : These hormones increase muscle tone. In hypothyroidism, skeletal muscles become weak and flabby.

- **GIT** : Thyroid hormones increase the motility of the GI tract.

THERAPEUTIC INDICATIONS:

Levothyroxine and liothyronine are the synthetic analogs of T4 and T3 respectively.

- **Cretinism** : This is hypothyroidism that occurs in infancy due to iodine deficiency or hypoplasia of the gland. Treatment must be instituted as soon as possible to avoid mental retardation.

- **Myxedema** : This is hypothyroidism that occurs in adults. It can occur due to autoimmune destruction of the gland, or surgical removal of the gland.

THYROID HORMONE INHIBITORS

Hyperthyroidism can occur due to an autoimmune disease called Grave's disease, or due to tumors of the thyroid gland. While surgical removal of all or part of the thyroid gland is the best option for the management of tumors, autoimmune conditions may be managed by thyroid hormone inhibitors. A few of the commonly used inhibitors are described below.

Drugs that inhibit synthesis of thyroid hormones
- This group includes propylthiouracil, methimazole, and carbimazole. They inhibit oxidation of iodine as well as coupling reactions. Propylthiouracil also inhibits the conversion of T4 to T3.
- These drugs can be taken orally, are metabolized in the liver and excreted in the urine. They cross the placenta and are secreted in breast milk. Prophylthiouracil has a short half-life of 1-2 hours, whereas carbimazole has a long half-life of 6-10 hours.
- These drugs are indicated in Grave's disease and toxic nodular goiter. They are also used preoperatively to bring the patient to the euthyroid state prior to removal of the gland.

- Adverse effects include loss of taste, GI intolerance, and liver damage. Fever, skin rashes, and joint pain have also been reported. Prolonged use of these drugs may lead to hypothyroidism.

Drugs that inhibit iodine trapping by thyroid cells

These drugs include thiocyanates, perchlorates, and nitrates. They act by blocking the sodium/iodide symporter (NIS) system. Although they have similar indications, these drugs are no longer used because of their high adverse effect profile. Thiocyanates can cause toxicity of the liver, brain, bone marrow, and kidney. Perchlorates have been linked to aplastic anemia and agranulocytosis.

Drugs that inhibit release of thyroid hormones

- Iodine and iodides tend to block the release of thyroid hormones. These drugs are effective for short-term use. After around ten days, the effect is lost, and excess hormones are released, leading to a toxic state.

- They are generally indicated for pre-operative control, and in emergencies like thyroid storm, to rapidly bring down thyroid levels.

Drugs that destroy thyroid cells

- Radioactive iodine is used to destroy thyroid cells from within. I^{131} emits radiation in the form of x-rays and beta particles. When this is ingested, it is preferentially taken up by the thyroid gland. The radiation causes necrosis of the thyroid cells.

- It is employed for diagnostic purposes, to detect 'hot spots' within the gland on scanning. It is also employed as a therapeutic measure in Grave's disease, toxic nodular goiter, and as palliative therapy in metastatic cancer of the thyroid gland.

Management of Thyroid Storm

Thyroid storm is an acute, toxic state of hyperthyroidism, where all the symptoms of this condition are exaggerated. The treatment regimen for this emergency must include the following:

- **Non-selective beta blockers** : These reduce peripheral conversion of T4 to T3. Control tachycardia.

- **Propylthiouracil** : Reduces the synthesis of thyroid hormone.

- **Iodine containing contrast media like iopanoic acid** : Inhibits release of hormones, as well as conversion of T4 to T3.

- **Corticosteroids** : May control concomitant adrenal crisis, provides symptomatic relief.

EXERCISES

1. When dietary iodine is taken up inside the cell, which ion is involved in its symporter?
   a. Potassium
   b. Sodium
   c. Calcium
   d. Chloride

2. How are synthetic thyroid hormones excreted?
   a. Urine
   b. Feces
   c. Bile
   d. Sweat

3. Which of the following metabolic processes is not mediated by thyroid hormones?
   a. Gluconeogenesis
   b. Glycogenesis
   c. Lipolysis
   d. Glycogenolysis

4. Which of the following is not a feature of hyperthyroid patients?
   a. Tachycardia
   b. Tremors
   c. Anemia
   d. Increased GI motility

5. What is the half-life of carbimazole?
   a. 1 to 2 hours
   b. 4 to 6 hours
   c. 6 to 10 hours
   d. 10 to 14 hours

6. Which of the following drugs has the potential to cause agranulocytosis?
    a. Thiocyanates
    b. Percolate
    c. Nitrate
    d. Iodide

7. Which of the following is not suitable for long-term control of hyperthyroidism?
    a. Propylthiouracil
    b. Methimazole
    c. Carbimazole
    d. Iodide

8. Which of the following is the commonly employed radioactive form of iodine?
    a. I-127
    b. I-129
    c. I-130
    d. I-131

9. Which drug is preferred for management of thyroid storm?
    a. Propylthiouracil
    b. Methimazole
    c. Carbimazole
    d. Thiocyanate

10. Which amino acid is involved in synthesis of thyroid hormone?
    a. Aspartate
    b. Glutamate
    c. Tyrosine
    d. Histidine

CHAPTER 5

Drugs Involved in Calcium and Bone Metabolism

Calcium plays a vital role in body functioning. It is an important intracellular component and also forms a major component of mineralized bone. Calcium metabolism is regulated by two important hormones in the body – the parathyroid hormone and calcitonin. This chapter discusses calcium, these hormones, and other drugs involved in bone metabolism.

CALCIUM

Physiological functions:
- Essential component of mineralized part of bone.
- Calcium excitation-coupling plays a role in muscle contraction, secretion from glands, and release of neurotransmitters.
- Serves as an intracellular messenger.
- Controls generation of electrical activity in the heart.
- Activation of clotting factors during the coagulation cascade.

Kinetics:
Calcium metabolism is regulated by a balanced interaction between three hormones – parathormone, calcitonin, and vitamin D (Calcitriol). Dietary calcium is absorbed from the small intestine. Usually, only about one-third of ingested calcium is absorbed. Around 40% of calcium binds to plasma proteins. It is excreted through the urine, but large amounts are reabsorbed. Unabsorbed calcium is also excreted through feces.

Therapeutic indications:
- Osteoporosis
- Increased requirements – children, pregnant and lactating women
- For acute treatment in tetany

PARATHYROID HORMONE:

Parathormone (PTH) is secreted by the parathyroid glands. The secretion is usually regulated by plasma calcium levels in an inverse fashion.

Physiological functions:

The overall effect of PTH is to increase plasma levels of calcium. This is achieved by:

- **Bone** : It increases osteoclastic activity, which promotes release of calcium from bone into the bloodstream. This encourages bone remodeling.
- **Kidney** : It increases calcium reabsorption from the distal convoluted tubule. It also activates the enzyme 1α hydroxylase, which converts dietary vitamin D into calcitriol. This indirectly increases plasma calcium levels.

CALCITONIN:

Calcitonin is produced by the parafollicular cells (C cells) of the thyroid gland. Its secretion is directly regulated by plasma calcium levels.

Physiological functions:

- Calcitonin functions as an antagonist to PTH, and decreases calcium levels in plasma.
- **Bone:** It inhibits osteoclastic activity and promotes bone deposition.
- **Kidney:** It inhibits reabsorption of calcium and phosphate from the proximal convoluted tubule.

Therapeutic indications:

Intranasal calcitonin is used to treat osteoporosis in post-menopausal women.

VITAMIN D:

Inactive vitamin D (Cholecalciferol) is usually synthesized in the skin, on exposure to sunlight. Under ideal conditions, dietary supplementation is not required, and this is therefore considered a hormone. Cholecalciferol is activated in the kidney to calcitriol, under the influence of the enzyme 1α hydroxylase.

Physiological functions:

- It promotes the absorption of calcium and phosphorus from the intestine.
- It promotes recruitment and differentiation of osteoclasts, which in turn promotes release of calcium and phosphorus from bone. It indirectly helps to maintain bone mineralization. If vitamin D levels fall, more PTH is secreted, which increases demineralization of bone. Therefore, bones become soft, and leads to rickets in children and osteomalacia in adults.
- It enhances reabsorption of calcium and phosphate from the kidney.

Pharmacokinetics:

Vitamin D3 is well absorbed from the intestines. It binds to plasma α-globulin in circulation, and is stored in the adipose tissue. When needed, it is activated to calcitriol. Calcitriol is metabolized in the liver, and metabolites are excreted in bile.

Therapeutic uses:

- Vitamin D deficiency (rickets, osteomalacia), or supplementation when there is an increased requirement (pregnant women).
- **Hypoparathyroidism**: It is preferred to administer PTH, in order to maintain calcium balance.
- **Osteoporosis**: It is more useful in preventing osteoporosis due to secondary hypoparathyroidism.

BISPHOSPHONATES

Bisphosphonates are a group of drugs that are used in the treatment of bone disorders.

Mechanism of action:

Bisphosphonates decrease osteoclastic activity and increase apoptosis of osteoclasts. This leads to an inhibition of bone resorption, which gradually increases bone mass.

Pharmacokinetics:

Bisphosphonates are not absorbed efficiently via the oral food, and absorption can be retarded by food or medication intake. Intravenous route is more effective. They are rapidly distributed to bone, where they persist for a long period of time. Elimination eventually occurs through the urine.

Adverse effects:

- Esophagitis, diarrhea, abdominal pain
- Musculoskeletal pain
- Long-term use may cause atypical fractures
- With high doses, osteonecrosis of the jaw has been reported

Indications:

The potency and indications of the different generations of bisphosphonates is summarized in Table 1.

Table 1. Potency and indications of bisphosphonates

GENERATION	DRUG NAME	POTENCY	INDICATIONS
First	Etidronate	1	Hypercalcemia
Second	Pamidronate	100	Osteoporosis
	Alendronate	500	Paget's disease
	Ibandronate	500	
Third	Risedronate	1000	Same as second-generation; when there is an increased severity of disease
	Zoledronate	5000	Hypercalcemia of malignancy
			Bone metastases

ESTROGEN RECEPTOR MODULATORS

- In post-menopausal women, estrogen efficiency can increase osteoclastic activity and decrease bone mass.
- Estrogen itself has several adverse effects. Therefore, drugs that interact with estrogen receptors are used.
- Raloxifene is an estrogen receptor modulator. It has agonist effects on bone, but antagonist effects on breast and endometrial tissue. Therefore, it can increase bone mass with minimum adverse effects.

EXERCISES

1. Which of the following is a physiological function of calcium?
    a. Intracellular messenger
    b. Bone mineral
    c. Role in muscle contraction
    d. All of the above

2. How much of dietary calcium is actually absorbed by the body?
    a. One-fourth
    b. One-thirds
    c. Two-thirds
    d. Five-eights

3. Which of the following is not a function of PTH?
    a. Increasing plasma calcium level
    b. Increasing osteoclastic activity in bone
    c. Promoting calcium reabsorption in kidney
    d. Promoting intestinal calcium absorption

4. Which of the following drugs is usually given in hypoparathyroidism?
    a. Vitamin D
    b. Parathormone
    c. Calcitonin
    d. Bisphosphonates

5. Which of the following endocrine glands secretes calcitonin?
    a. Thyroid
    b. Parathyroid
    c. Pituitary
    d. Thymus

6. Which of the following routes of administration is preferred for calcitonin?
   a. Oral
   b. Intranasal
   c. Intramuscular
   d. Rectal

7. Which of the following forms of vitamin D is synthesized in the skin?
   a. Ergocalciferol
   b. Calciferol
   c. Cholecalciferol
   d. Calcitriol

8. Which of the following bisphosphonate drugs is used for treatment of bone metastases?
   a. Etidronate
   b. Pamidronate
   c. Alendronate
   d. Zoledronate

9. What is the potency of risedronate as compared to etidronate?
   a. 50
   b. 100
   c. 1000
   d. 5000

10. On which of the following tissues does raloxifene have an agonist effect?
    a. Breast
    b. Bone
    c. Endometrium
    d. All of the above

CHAPTER 6

Insulin and Oral Hypoglycemic Drugs

Insulin is a hormone that is secreted by the beta cells of the islets of the pancreas. It is primarily concerned with glucose metabolism.

Diabetes mellitus is a disease that is characterized by deficiency in the supply or functioning of insulin. This is one of the most common diseases affecting people worldwide. Classically, there are two types of diabetes:

- **Type 1 diabetes** : In this condition, the beta cells of the pancreatic islets are destroyed due to viruses or toxins. This leads to an absolute lack of insulin, and can only be treated by replacing insulin. This type affects children and adolescents and is therefore called 'juvenile diabetes'.

- **Type 2 diabetes** : This disease commonly affects older adults. While the beta cells of the pancreas are functioning, there is peripheral resistance to insulin and the target organs fail to take up insulin. Over a period of time, the apparent decreased requirement by the target organs cause the beta cell function to decline, and may eventually result in an actual insulin deficit.

INSULIN AND INSULIN ANALOGS

Insulin is an anabolic hormone that converts glucose, amino acids, and fatty acids to glycogen, proteins, and lipids.

Physiological functions:

- Promotes transport of glucose across the cell membrane of cells like skeletal muscle and fat.
- It promotes glycogenesis in the liver, and inhibits gluconeogenesis.
- In adipose tissue, it promotes triglyceride synthesis and inhibits lipolysis. It also increases levels of the enzyme lipoprotein lipase, which helps in clearing chylomicrons and very low-density lipoprotein (VLDL).
- It promotes protein synthesis from amino acids and prevents protein breakdown.

151

To replace the deficiency of insulin in diabetes, synthetic insulin is used. This is obtained from genetically altered strains of microorganisms like E.coli and yeast, using recombinant DNA technology. Depending on the amino acid sequence used, insulins having different properties can be produced.

Synthetic preparations of insulin:

Depending on the onset and duration of action, the preparations are classified as rapid-acting, short-acting, intermediate-acting, and long-acting preparations. These drugs are summarized in Table 1.

Table 1. Classification of different insulin preparations.

TYPE OF PREPARATION	EXAMPLES	ONSET OF ACTION (HOURS)	DURATION OF ACTION (HOURS)	INDICATIONS
Rapid-acting	Insulin lispro Insulin aspart Insulin glulisine	0.2 to 0.4	3 to 5	Control of postprandial glucose (functions like mealtime insulin) Emergency treatment of uncomplicated diabetic ketoacidosis
Short-acting	Regular insulin	0.5 to 1	6 to 8	May be combined with longer acting insulins to control fasting glucose levels Used for emergency control of blood glucose levels
Intermediate-acting	Insulin zinc suspension (Lente insulin) Neutral protamine hagedorn (NPH insulin)	1 to 2	8 to 10	Basal control of blood glucose levels in Type I diabetics
Long-acting	Insulin glargine Insulin detemir	2 to 4	20 to 24	Basal control of blood glucose levels in Type I diabetics

Pharmacokinetics:

Synthetic insulin cannot be given orally as it gets degraded in the GIT. It is usually administered as subcutaneous injections. Both natural and synthetic insulin are metabolized largely in the liver. Some metabolism also occurs in the skeletal muscle and kidney.

Adverse effects:

- Hypoglycemia
- Lipodystrophy at the injection site

152

• Weight gain

ORAL HYPOGLYCEMIC DRUGS

These drugs are used for the management of Type 2 diabetes. They are more popular for management as they can be taken orally, unlike insulin, which must be injected.

SULFONYLUREAS

These drugs promote the release of insulin from the pancreas. They are classified as first-generation drugs (tolbutamide, chlorpropamide) and second-generation drugs (glimepiride, glipizide, glyburide). The second-generation drugs are more potent, and have a better pharmacological profile. They have completely replaced first-generation drugs.

Mechanism of action:

These drugs block ATP-sensitive potassium channels in the islet cells. This causes depolarization, which in turn leads to calcium influx, and exocytosis of insulin. They also improve the sensitivity of the target cells to insulin.

Pharmacokinetics:

These drugs are well absorbed by the oral route, and are highly bound to plasma proteins. Metabolism occurs in the liver, and the drug is excreted in urine and feces. The half-life of different sulfonylureas is as follows:

• Glyburide 2 to 4 hours
• Glipizide – 3 to 5 hours
• Glimepiride – 5 to 7 hours
• Gliclazide 8 to 20 hours

Adverse effects:

• **Hypoglycemia** : Patients with liver and kidney dysfunction, and elderly patients are especially susceptible.
• **Renal dysfunction** : The risk is especially high with glyburide.
• **Hypersensitivity reactions** : May cause flushing and skin rashes.

MEGLITINIDE ANALOGS

These drugs have a quick onset and short duration of action. The drugs repaglinide and nateglinide belong to this category.

Mechanism of action:

Like sulfonylureas, these drugs also act on ATP-sensitive potassium channels and stimulate insulin secretion. As compared to sulfonylureas, they act quickly and for a short period of time. They stimulate insulin in response to food, and are effective at postprandial blood glucose control.

Pharmacokinetics:

They are well absorbed orally, and must be taken prior to meals for effective glucose control. Metabolism occurs through the cytochrome P450 system of the liver, and excretion occurs through bile.

Adverse effects:

- **Hypoglycemia**: they must never be combined with sulfonylureas as this potentiates the risk.
- Minor side effects: headache, arthralgia, weight gain

BIGUANIDES

The only biguanide that is therapeutically used today is metformin. It is the drug of choice for initial therapy in Type 2 diabetes. Apart from diabetes, it is also used to improve insulin sensitivity in polycystic ovary disease.

Mechanism of action:

Metformin increases the sensitivity of target organs to insulin. It reduces intestinal absorption of glucose and inhibits hepatic gluconeogenesis. It also improves utilization of glucose by peripheral tissues.

Pharmacokinetics:

The drug is well absorbed through the oral route. It does not bind to any plasma proteins, and does not undergo metabolism. It is excreted unchanged through the urine.

Adverse effects and contraindications:

- **Minor GIT effects**: Abdominal pain, metallic taste, bloating, anorexia, and diarrhea.
- Contraindicated in patients with renal dysfunction as they can develop lactic acidosis.
- It must be discontinued if the patient develops conditions that predispose to renal failure, such as myocardial infarction, cardiac failure, and sepsis. It must also be temporarily withdrawn in patients receiving contrast dye for CT scans, as the dye is nephrotoxic.

THIAZOLIDINEDIONES:

Pioglitazone and rosiglitazone are the drugs in this category. They are also used in the treatment of polycystic ovary disease.

Mechanism of action

These drugs are agonists for a specific nuclear receptor called peroxisome proliferator-activated receptor-γ (PPAR-γ). Binding to this receptor stimulates the transcription of genes that increase insulin sensitivity. This action takes place in the adipose tissue, liver, and skeletal muscle.

Pharmacokinetics:

These drugs are well absorbed through the oral route, and are highly bound to serum albumin. Metabolism occurs in the liver through the cytochrome P450 system. While pioglitazone is largely excreted through the feces, rosiglitazone is excreted through urine.

Adverse effects:

- Has the potential to cause liver toxicity.
- **Minor side effects**: Weight gain due to increase in subcutaneous fat and fluid retention.
- Long-term pioglitazone use may increase the risk of bladder cancer.
- Rosiglitazone is banned in a few countries because of the high risk of myocardial infarction and stroke.

α-GLUCOSIDASE INHIBITORS

These drugs, including acarbose, voglibose, and miglitol, are used for the control of postprandial blood glucose levels.

Mechanism of action:

As the name suggests, these drugs inhibit the enzyme α-glucosidase. They retard the digestion of carbohydrates. This prevents glucose absorption and lowers blood glucose levels.

Pharmacokinetics:

Acarbose is poorly absorbed through the oral route, while miglitol is well absorbed. The drugs are metabolized by intestinal bacteria, and metabolites are excreted through urine.

Adverse effects:

- They can cause abdominal cramps, flatulence, and diarrhea.
- These drugs are not indicated in patients with pre-existing GIT conditions like ulcers, inflammatory bowel disease, or intestinal obstruction.

DIPEPTIDYL-PEPTIDASE INHIBITORS:

These drugs stimulate secretion of insulin and include the drugs sitagliptin, saxagliptin, alogliptin, and linagliptin.

Mechanism of action:

Dipeptidyl peptidase is an enzyme that degrades an incretin hormone, GLP-1, which increases insulin secretion in response to meals. By inhibiting the degrading enzyme, the life of GLP-1 is prolonged, and this enhances insulin secretion.

Pharmacokinetics:

They are well absorbed through the oral route, and are unaffected by food intake. Saxagliptin undergoes metabolism in the liver through the cytochrome P450 system, and is excreted in the urine. Sitagliptin and alogliptin are excreted unchanged in the urine, while linagliptin is excreted out through the enterohepatic system.

Adverse effects:

- **Minor effects**: Headache, nasopharyngitis
- Pancreatitis is a rare but serious adverse effect.

SODIUM GLUCOSE COTRANSPORTER-2 INHIBITORS

This is a newer category of drugs, and had two important agents – canagliflozin and dapagliflozin.

Mechanism of action:

The sodium glucose cotransporter-2 system is responsible for reabsorbing glucose into the blood at the proximal tubule of the kidney. Inhibiting this transporter system results in glycosuria, and decrease in blood glucose levels. This drug, however, also decreases sodium reabsorption, and may cause osmotic diuresis.

Pharmacokinetics:

Absorption is through oral route and is optimal on an empty stomach. They are metabolized in the liver by glucuronide conjugation. Excretion occurs through urine and feces.

Adverse effects:

- Increases susceptibility to genital fungal infections and urinary tract infections, particularly in women.
- Increased frequency of urination
- Hypotension may occur due to an increased urine output.

EXERCISES

1. What is the duration of action of insulin glulisine?
   a. 3 to 5 hours
   b. 6 to 10 hours
   c. 10-14 hours
   d. 20 to 24 hours

2. What is the preferred route of administration of insulin?
   a. Oral
   b. Intramuscular
   c. Subcutaneous
   d. Rectal

3. Which ion channels are blocked by the use of sulfonylureas?
   a. Sodium
   b. Potassium
   c. Calcium
   d. Chloride

4. Which of the following sulfonylureas has the longest plasma half-life?
   a. Glyburide
   b. Glipizide
   c. Glimepiride
   d. Gliclazide

5. Which of the following sulfonylureas has the highest risk of renal dysfunction?
   a. Glyburide
   b. Glipizide
   c. Glimepiride
   d. Gliclazide

6. Which of the following oral hypoglycemic drugs has a high risk of bladder cancer?
   a. Repaglinide
   b. Pioglitazone
   c. Rosiglitazone
   d. Metformin

7. Which of the following drugs is the first-line drug in diabetes mellitus?
   a. Acarbose
   b. Sitagliptin
   c. Canagliflozin
   d. Metformin

8. Which of the following oral hypoglycemic drugs acts by preventing digestion of carbohydrates?
   a. Sitagliptin
   b. Miglitol
   c. Tolbutamide
   d. Nateglinide

9. Which of the following drugs can cause nasopharyngitis?
   a. Acarbose
   b. Sitagliptin
   c. Metformin
   d. Pioglitazone

10. Which of the following oral hypoglycemic drugs promote diuresis?
    a. Acarbose
    b. Sitagliptin
    c. Canagliflozin
    d. Metformin

CHAPTER 7

Corticosteroids

The adrenal gland secretes two main kinds of hormones. The inner adrenal medulla secretes catecholamines, namely adrenaline and noradrenaline. These have already been discussed in the chapter on adrenergic drugs. The outer adrenal cortex secretes corticosteroids and adrenal androgens. The current chapter focuses on corticosteroids.

There are two types of corticosteroids, glucocorticoids and mineralocorticoids. The outer part of the adrenal cortex, called the zona glomerulosa, secretes mineralocorticoids. The middle part, zona fasciculata, synthesizes glucocorticoids. The inner part of the adrenal cortex, called the zona reticularis, secretes adrenal androgens.

MINERALOCORTICOIDS

The main mineralocorticoid in the body is aldosterone.

Physiological functions:

- Enhances reabsorption of sodium in the distal convoluted tubule of the kidney.
- Enhances concomitant excretion of potassium and hydrogen ions.
- It also enhances reabsorption of sodium from other parts of the body such as the gastrointestinal mucosa, sweat and salivary glands.

GLUCOCORTICOIDS

The main glucocorticoid produced in the human body is cortisol. It is produced upon stimulation from corticotropin-releasing hormone (CRH) and adrenocorticotropic hormone (ACTH) from the hypothalamus and pituitary gland, and has a negative feedback relationship with these structures.

Physiological functions:

- They promote catabolism of proteins and lipolysis. They also promote gluconeogenesis from amino acids and fatty acids.
- They provide excess glucose needed in cases of stress, trauma, and infection.

- They increase blood levels of red blood cells, neutrophils, and platelets. They decrease blood levels of eosinophils, basophils, lymphocytes, and monocytes. The overall effect is immunosuppression.
- They exert anti-inflammatory activity by inhibiting the enzyme phospholipase A2. This enzyme is responsible for the release of arachidonic acid, which is the precursor of pro-inflammatory prostaglandins and leukotrienes.
- They decrease blood calcium levels by inhibiting intestinal absorption and promoting renal excretion of calcium ions.
- Glucocorticoids help maintain normal glomerular filtration in the kidney and enhance tubular secretion.

SYNTHETIC CORTICOSTEROIDS

Synthetic corticosteroids have different levels of mineralocorticoid and glucocorticoid activity. The commonest steroid used is hydrocortisone, and it is taken as a reference drug against which the potency of other drugs is compared.

Table 1: Potency and indications of different corticosteroids.

CATEGORY	DURATION OF ACTION	DRUG NAME	POTENCY - MINERALO- CORTICOID FUNCTION	POTENCY - GLUCO- CORTICOID FUNCTION	SPECIFIC INDICATIONS
Reference	Short-acting	Hydrocortisone	1	1	Acute adrenal insufficiency Status asthmaticus Shock
Mostly glucocorticoid function	Intermediate-acting drugs	Prednisolone Methylprednisolone	0.8 0.5	4 5	Autoimmune diseases Transplant patients
Mostly mineralocorticoid function	Long-acting drugs	Triamcinolone Dexamethasone Betamethasone	0 0 0	5 25 25	Mostly topical use Inflammation, allergies, shock, cerebral edema
		Desoxycorticosterone acetate Fludrocortisone	100 150	10 0.3	Addison's disease

Pharmacokinetics:

Most synthetic corticosteroids are well absorbed orally. Some are also available for intramuscular or intravenous injection. Corticosteroids are also available as topical ointments and intranasal sprays, and some amount gets absorbed systemically through this route. More than 90% of absorbed corticosteroids are bound to plasma albumin or globulin. They are metabolized in the liver through oxidation and glucuronide conjugation. Excretion occurs through the urine.

Therapeutic indications:

- **Primary adrenal insufficiency (Addison's disease)** : Fludrocortisone is the preferred drug.

- **Secondary and tertiary adrenal insufficiency** : It can occur due to ACTH and CRH suppression. This is often seen in patients who take long-term steroids. Hydrocortisone is preferred.

- **Inflammation** : They are useful in reducing swelling due to surgery in the postoperative period. They are also used for long-term management in inflammatory conditions like arthritis.

- **Allergic conditions** : Asthma, allergic rhinitis benefit from intranasal inhalation of steroids.

- **Lung maturation** : In the fetus, cortisol promotes lung maturation. Steroids are used to accelerate lung maturation in premature infants.

Adverse effects:

These are dose-dependent and are more common in patients who are on long-term therapy.

- **Osteoporosis** : Due to decreased calcium levels
- **Hyperglycemia** : Glycemic control is worsened in diabetics
- Impaired wound healing and increased risk of infection
- **Minor effects**: Increased appetite, emotional disturbances, and weight gain in the central region of the body.
- **Secondary adrenal insufficiency**: This can develop if the patient abruptly discontinues the drugs, or there is an increased steroid requirement in times of stress. Endogenous steroid production is suppressed due to exogenous suppression of CRH and ACTH.

GLUCOCORTICOID INHIBITORS:

Certain drugs can suppress the synthesis and function of glucocorticoids. These are drugs that were primarily developed for other purposes, and their properties are discussed in detail in the relevant chapters.

Ketoconazole:

- This is an antifungal agent.
- It inhibits synthesis of hormones both from the adrenal gland and gonadal hormones.
- It is used in therapy of Cushing's syndrome (excess steroid production by the adrenal gland).

Spironolactone:

- This is a competitive antagonist for the mineralocorticoid receptor in the kidney. It also antagonizes the synthesis of aldosterone and testosterone. Therefore, it reduces reabsorption of sodium in the kidney.
- It is used in congestive heart failure, and to manage hirsutism in women.
- Adverse effects include skin rashes, gynecomastia, dysmenorrhea, and rarely, hyperkalemia.

Eplerenone:

- This is also an aldosterone antagonist, and binds to the mineralocorticoid receptor.
- Also used in heart failure and hypertension. Unlike spironolactone, it does not cause gynecomastia.

EXERCISES

1. Which part of the adrenal gland is responsible for the release of glucocorticoids?
   a. Adrenal medulla
   b. Zona glomerulosa
   c. Zona fasciculata
   d. Zona reticularis

2. Sodium reabsorption occurs from all the following body parts except:
   a. Proximal convoluted tubule
   b. Distal convoluted tubule
   c. Salivary glands
   d. Gastrointestinal mucosa

3. Which of the following is not an indication for corticosteroid therapy?
   a. Allergic rhinitis
   b. Rheumatoid arthritis
   c. Osteoporosis
   d. Addison's disease

4. Which of the following corticosteroids is indicated for treatment of Addison's disease?
   a. Hydrocortisone
   b. Fludrocortisone
   c. Prednisolone
   d. Dexamethasone

5. Which of the following corticosteroids is preferred in management of acute asthmatic attacks?
   a. Hydrocortisone
   b. Fludrocortisone
   c. Prednisolone
   d. Dexamethasone

6. Which of the following corticosteroids has the maximum potency?
   a. Hydrocortisone
   b. Fludrocortisone
   c. Prednisolone
   d. Dexamethasone

7. As compared to hydrocortisone, what is the potency of prednisolone?
   a. 3 times
   b. 4 times
   c. 5 times
   d. 6 times

8. Which of the following antifungal agents inhibits corticosteroid synthesis?
   a. Fluconazole
   b. Ketoconazole
   c. Miconazole
   d. Itraconazole

9. What is the risk of giving corticosteroids in the postoperative period?
   a. Impaired pain tolerance
   b. Increase of swelling
   c. Impaired wound healing
   d. Increased bleeding from wound

10. Which of the side effects of spironolactone is eliminated by the use of eplerenone?
    a. Skin rashes
    b. Dysmenorrhea
    c. Gynecomastia
    d. Hyperkalemia

CHAPTER 8

Androgens, Estrogens and Progestins

These hormones are also referred to as gonadal or sex hormones. They are primarily involved in pubertal maturation and reproduction.

ANDROGENS

Androgens are a group of sex hormones that have masculinizing effects. In the males, the predominant androgenic hormone is testosterone, which is secreted by the Leydig cells of the testes. In females, some secretion occurs in the ovaries, and some secretion occurs from adrenal gland in both genders.

Synthetic androgens include methyltestosterone and fluoxymesterone. They are not as effective as testosterone, but have better bioavailability. Certain synthetic androgens have higher anabolic and lower androgenic activity. They are referred to as anabolic steroids, and include drugs like oxymetholone, methandienone, and nandrolone.

Physiological actions:
- Promotes growth of male genital organs during puberty.
- Promotes development of male secondary sexual characteristics, including facial, pubic, and axillary hair growth. This also includes growth of larynx and deepening of voice.
- Induces pubertal growth spurt, which allows for growth of the skeleton and skeletal muscles.
- Promotes erythropoiesis, which increases the hematocrit of men relative to women.

Pharmacokinetics:
Natural testosterone undergoes high first-pass metabolism in the liver. They must be combined with esterified lipids to increase the bioavailability and duration of action. However, synthetic androgens are metabolized slowly and have a much longer duration of action. In plasma, androgens are highly bound to plasma proteins.

Metabolism occurs in the liver, mostly through glucuronide conjugation. Excretion occurs through the urine.

Adverse effects:
- In females, androgens can cause hirsutism, deepening of voice, and male pattern baldness.
- In males, excessive use of androgens can cause priapism, gynecomastia, and impotence.
- Anabolic steroid use can cause premature closure of epiphyseal plates, causing stunted growth. They can also cause mood disturbances and aggression.

Therapeutic uses:
- Testosterone is usually used for the treatment of primary or secondary hypogonadism.
- Anabolic steroids are used to treat muscle wasting in conditions like AIDS or cancer. Moreover, they may also be used to treat senile osteoporosis and severe burns.
- Androgens can be used to enhance skeletal growth in prepubertal boys with pituitary dwarfism.

ANTI-ANDROGENS
- These are a group of drugs that block the synthesis or actions of androgens.
- Finasteride and dutasteride block synthesis of testosterone by inhibiting the enzyme 5-α-reductase.
- Flutamide, nilutamide, and related drugs compete with androgens for their receptors and block their effects.
- These drugs find application in treatment of benign prostate hyperplasia, or in prostate cancer.

ESTROGENS
Estrogens are a group of hormones that are secreted by the ovary. The principal estrogen is estradiol. Estrone and estriol are metabolites of estradiol and are less potent.

Physiological functions:
- Brings about pubertal changes in women such as growth of uterus, ovaries, and fallopian tubes.
- Confers secondary sexual characteristics, such as development of breasts, pubic and axillary hair.

- Maintains bone mass by preventing bone resorption and increasing the expression of bone matrix proteins.

- **Metabolic effects**: Estrogens decrease plasma low-density lipoprotein (LDL) and cholesterol, and increase high-density lipoprotein (HDL) and triglyceride levels. They may slightly impair glucose tolerance.

- **Blood vessels**: They increase blood coagulability and fibrinolytic activity. They also relax vessel wall musculature and cause vasodilation.

Types of therapeutic estrogens:

- **Natural** : Estradiol is predominantly used. It is not very effective when taken orally.

- **Synthetic estrogens** : These include steroidal derivatives like ethinyl estradiol, and non-steroidal derivatives like diethylstilbestrol.

Pharmacokinetics:

Estradiol is rapidly absorbed through the skin, mucous membranes, and GIT. However, from the GIT, it is immediately metabolized by the liver. Synthetic compounds are well absorbed orally, and are stored in the adipose tissue, from which they are released slowly. They are metabolized both in the liver and peripheral tissues. They are excreted in the bile, and active metabolites are reabsorbed through enterohepatic circulation. Inactive metabolites are eventually excreted through the urine.

Adverse effects:

- **Minor effects** – Nausea, breast tenderness, migraine
- Increased risk of breast and endometrial cancer, especially with unopposed use (without progestin).
- Increased risk of thromboembolic events such as myocardial infarction.

Therapeutic uses:

- **Post-menopausal hormonal replacement therapy** : Menopause may cause unpleasant symptoms such as hot flushes, cognitive changes, and urogenital atrophy. Hormone replacement therapy can suppress these effects. However, due to the risk of adverse effects, the minimum possible dose of estrogen must be used.

- **Contraception** : For this purpose, it is usually used in combination with progesterone.

ESTROGEN RECEPTOR MODULATORS

These are drugs that have either agonist or antagonist effects on estrogen receptors.

Clinical actions:

- **Antagonist effects in breast tissue** : Tamoxifen, toremifene, and raloxifene are competitive antagonists for estrogen in the breast tissue.

- **Agonist effect on bone** : Raloxifene acts similar to estrogen in preserving bone mass.

- **Endometrium** : Tamoxifen can act like estrogen and predispose to endometrial cancer. Raloxifene does not have agonist activity in this region.

- **Metabolic effects** : Like estrogen, raloxifene lowers LDL and cholesterol levels in plasma.

- **Influence on pituitary** : Some drugs like clomiphene are only partial agonists, and interfere with the negative feedback mechanism on the pituitary. This increases secretion of gonadotropin-releasing hormone, which in turn stimulates gonadotropin secretion and stimulates ovulation.

Pharmacokinetics:

These drugs are absorbed orally. Metabolism occurs in the liver through cytochrome P450 system and glucuronide conjugation. Metabolites are excreted in the bile, undergo enterohepatic circulation, and are finally excreted through feces.

Adverse effects:

Estrogen modulator inhibitor	Adverse effects
Tamoxifene	Hot flashes, nausea, endometrial hyperplasia and malignancy
Raloxifene	Hot flashes, nausea, Increased risk of thromboembolic events
Clomiphene	Headache, nausea, hot flushes, Ovarian enlargement, risk of multiple births

Therapeutic uses:

- **Tamoxifen** – Metastatic breast cancer to reduce malignancy size
- **Raloxifene** – Prevention of osteoporosis in post-menopausal women
- **Clomiphene** – Infertility due to anovulation
- **Ospemifene** – Treatment of dyspareunia

PROGESTOGENS

This hormone is secreted in response to stimulation from luteinizing hormone. It is secreted from the corpus luteum in the second half of the menstrual cycle, and also from the placenta. Small amounts are also secreted from the adrenal cortex, in both men and women.

Physiological functions:

- Progesterone basically primes the body for pregnancy.
- **Uterus**: It prepares the uterus for implantation. When progesterone levels decrease, menstruation occurs.
- **Vagina and cervix**: It thickens secretions, increases leukocyte infiltration.
- **Breast**: Prepares breast for lactation. Proliferation of acinar cells occurs.
- **Synthetic progesterones**: Natural progestin is not suitable for metabolic use, as it is metabolized rapidly. Some of the common synthetic progesterone derivatives include desogestrel, norethindrone, and medroxyprogesterone.

Pharmacokinetics:

Natural progesterone is metabolized rapidly when taken orally, and has a very short half-life. Synthetic progesterones can mostly be taken orally. They are metabolized slowly in the liver, and excreted in urine as inactive metabolites.

Adverse effects:

- Headache, breast tenderness, amenorrhea
- Long-term use can predispose to diabetes and breast cancer.

Therapeutic uses:

- Along with estrogen, it may be used in:
  - o Hormone replacement therapy for post-menopausal women
  - o For contraception
- **Dysmenorrhea**
- **Endometriosis: prevents bleeding from ectopic sites**
- **To prevent abortion in high-risk cases**

ANTI-PROGESTINS

- Mifepristone, an anti-progestin, has partial agonist-antagonist activity.
- It inhibits progesterone, and can thus be used to induce abortion in early pregnancy.
- **Adverse effect**: It can cause severe uterine bleeding.

EXERCISES

1. What is the main reason for using synthetic androgens and estrogens for therapeutic use?
   a. Natural forms are difficult to obtain
   b. Natural forms get metabolized very fast
   c. Natural forms are not absorbed well orally
   d. Natural forms may be toxic

2. Which drug is used in muscle wasting conditions?
   a. Mifepristone
   b. Desogestrel
   c. Nandrolone
   d. Tamoxifene

3. Which of the following drugs inhibits the synthesis of androgens?
   a. Finasteride
   b. Flutamide
   c. Mifepristone
   d. Raloxifene

4. Which of the following drugs is used to reduce the size of breast malignancies?
   a. Mifepristone
   b. Desogestrel
   c. Nandrolone
   d. Tamoxifene

5. Which of the following drugs is used for prevention of abortion?
   a. Mifepristone
   b. Desogestrel
   c. Nandrolone
   d. Tamoxifene

6. Which of the following drugs carries the risk of inducing multiple births?
    a. Tamoxifen
    b. Raloxifene
    c. Clomiphene
    d. Ospemifene

7. Which of the following drugs does not compete for estrogen in the breast tissue?
    a. Tamoxifen
    b. Raloxifene
    c. Clomiphene
    d. Ospemifene

8. Which of the following drugs is used for the treatment of dyspareunia?
    a. Tamoxifen
    b. Raloxifene
    c. Clomifene
    d. Ospemifene

9. Which of the following hormones primes the body for pregnancy?
    a. Estrogen
    b. Prolactin
    c. Progesterone
    d. Oxytocin

10. Which of the following drugs is used to induce abortion?
    a. Mifepristone
    b. Desogestrel
    c. Nandrolone
    d. Tamoxifene

UNIT VI : THE CARDIOVASCULAR SYSTEM

CHAPTER 1

Drugs Used in Hypertension

Antihypertensives are a group of drugs that are used to manage high blood pressure. Any patient who has systolic blood pressure above 140mmHg, or diastolic pressure above 90mmHg is considered to be hypertensive. Most patients suffer from primary or 'essential' hypertension, where the cause is not known. While hypertension itself does not cause any symptoms, it is a major risk factor in the development of other morbid conditions such as heart disease, stroke, and kidney failure.

There are several different categories of anti-hypertensive agents based on their mechanism of action. These drugs are chosen based on the degree of hypertension and other medical comorbidities present.

DIURETICS

The exact mechanism and pharmacology of diuretics is discussed in detail in Unit X. Basically, by promoting urinary excretion, diuretics decrease blood volume, which in turn lowers the blood pressure. Given in low doses, diuretics are the initial drug of choice for hypertension in most patients. The following forms of diuretics are used in the management of hypertension:

Thiazide diuretics:

- These include the drugs hydrochlorothiazide and chlorthalidone.
- These drugs lower blood pressure by increasing sodium and water excretion.
- Long-term use tends to normalize plasma volume. However, the hypotensive effect continues because of lowered peripheral vascular resistance.
- **Adverse effects**: Hypokalemia, hyperuricemia, hyperglycemia
- **Indications**: As monotherapy in patients with mild hypertension. May be combined with other drugs for moderate to severe hypertension.
- **Contraindications**: Cannot be used in patients with renal dysfunction (efficacy is reduced).

Loop diuretics:

- These include the drugs furosemide, bumetanide, and ethacrynic acid.
- They block sodium and chloride reabsorption in the kidney. They also increase renal blood flow and decrease renal peripheral vascular resistance.
- **Adverse effects**: Hypokalemia, fluid imbalance, hypercalcemia
- **Indications**: For management of hypertension in patients with

  o Congestive cardiac failure – decreases fluid load in these patients
  o Renal dysfunction

Potassium-sparing diuretics:

- These include the drugs triamterene, amiloride, and spironolactone.
- The first two drugs prevent sodium reabsorption, while spironolactone acts as an antagonist for aldosterone.
- They reduce potassium loss in urine and are therefore combined with the previous diuretics to prevent hypokalemia.

ACE INHIBITORS

The first angiotensin-converting enzyme inhibitor to be used was captopril. Today, commonly used drugs include enalapril and lisinopril.

Mechanism of action:

An important factor in the determination of blood pressure is the renin-angiotensin-aldosterone mechanism:

- The kidneys respond to decreased blood arterial pressure by releasing an enzyme called renin.
- Renin acts on angiotensinogen to convert it into angiotensin I.
- Angiotensin I is converted into angiotensin II in the presence of angiotensin converting enzyme (ACE).
- Angiotensin II causes vasoconstriction, which increases the blood pressure. It also stimulates secretion of aldosterone, which reabsorbs sodium and water, and increases the blood volume, thereby contributing to a rise in blood pressure.

ACE inhibitors prevent conversion of angiotensin I into angiotensin II. They reduce peripheral vascular resistance. Decreasing sodium and water retention also decreases the blood volume, which decreases the preload and after-load on the heart.

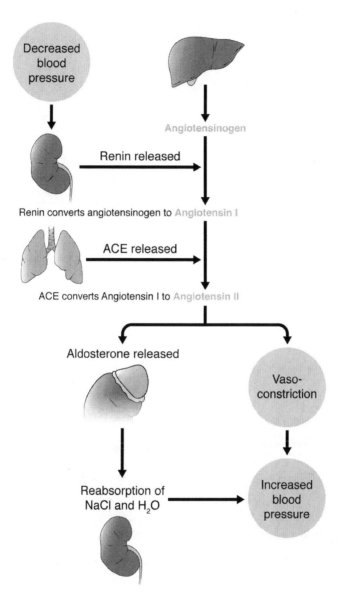

Figure 9 *The renin-angiotensin-aldosterone system is a hormone system within the body that is essential for the regulation of blood pressure and fluid balance. Kidneys respond to decreased blood pressure by releasing renin, which acts on angiotensinogen and converts it into angiotensin I. Angiotensin I is converted into angiotensin II in the presence of ACE. Angiotensin II causes vasoconstriction, thereby increasing blood pressure; it also stimulates secretion of aldosterone from the adrenal glands, which reabsorbs sodium and water, also contributing to the rise in blood pressure.*

Pharmacokinetics:

All ACE inhibitors can be taken orally. Metabolism generally occurs in the liver. For captopril and lisinopril, even the metabolites are active, so they may be preferred in patients with renal impairment. Most drug metabolites are excreted in the urine. The metabolites of fosinopril may be partly excreted through bile. The t1/2 of some ACE inhibitors is summarized in Table 1.

Table 1. Elimination half-life of ACE inhibitors

DRUG	ELIMINATION HALF-LIFE
Captopril	2 hours
Enalapril	11 hours
Lisinopril	12 hours
Fosinopril	12 hours
Perindopril	24 hours
Ramipril	48 hours

Adverse effects:

- **Minor**: Dry cough, fever, altered taste, headache, nausea
- Hypotension
- Rash, urticaria, angioedema: Due to increases bradykinin levels
- Hyperkalemia: Must not be combined with potassium-sparing diuretics
- Teratogen

Indications:

- **Hypertension** : May be used as first-line drugs for management of hypertension.
- **Congestive cardiac failure** : They decrease blood volume and reduce the workload on the heart.
- **Myocardial infarction** : ACE inhibitors reduce mortality following MI, if they are administered when MI is evolving, and are continued for up to six weeks.
- **Diabetic nephropathy** : It can prevent or delay end stage renal disease in diabetics.

ANGIOTENSIN II RECEPTOR BLOCKERS

- This category includes drugs such as losartan, candesartan, and olmesartan. These drugs block angiotensin II from binding to its receptors, thus inhibiting its functions.
- Like ACE inhibitors, they reduce blood volume by preventing salt and water reabsorption. They also lower peripheral vascular resistance.

- They do not decrease bradykinin levels and thus have a low risk of urticaria and angioedema.
- Their other adverse effects, and indications are similar to ACE inhibitors.
- They must not be combined with ACE inhibitors because of a similar adverse effect profile, which can be potentiated.

RENIN INHIBITOR

- Aliskiren is a drug that inhibits renin. It thus functions similar to ACE inhibitors and angiotensin receptor blockers. It should not be combined with these drug categories.
- It may be administered orally, but has low bioavailability. It is excreted in feces. Plasma half-life is 24 hours.

CALCIUM CHANNEL BLOCKERS

Mechanism of action:

Calcium basically mediates action potential development, and muscle contraction in smooth muscles and cardiac muscles. Calcium channel blockers (CCBs) prevent intracellular influx of calcium, which decreases the intracellular calcium and prevents action potential.

Clinical actions:

- **Smooth muscle relaxation** : This includes smooth muscle of the vascular walls, which causes vasodilation. This effect is mainly seen in arterioles, and not the veins.

- **Negative inotropic, chronotropic, and dromotropic action on the heart** : This means a decrease in the force of contraction, heart rate, and conduction velocity of the heart.

Pharmacokinetics:

Based on their chemical structure and pharmacokinetics, CCBs are divided into three categories:

- **Diphenylalkylamines** : Verapamil is the main drug in this category. It is well absorbed orally, and has a bioavailability of 15-30% due to high first-pass metabolism. It is metabolized in the liver and excreted in the urine. Plasma half-life is 4 to 6 hours.

- **Benzothiazepines** : This consists of one drug, diltiazem. It is well absorbed orally, has a bioavailability of 40% to 60%, and is 80% bound to plasma proteins. It is metabolized in the liver and excreted through urine. Plasma half-life is 5 to 6 hours.

- **Dihydropyridines** : This consists of several useful drugs, including nifedipine, amlodipine, and nicardipine. The pharmacokinetics are similar to the above drugs. Plasma half-life differs, with nifedipine having a short half-life of 2 to 5 hours, and amlodipine having the longest, ranging from 25 to 35 hours.

Adverse effects:

- **Verapamil** : Can cause constipation. It can also aggravate first degree AV block and is contraindicated in these conditions.

- **Dihydropyridines** : Dizziness, headache, fatigue, and peripheral edema. They can also cause gingival hyperplasia.

Indications:

- **Hypertension** : May be used both as first-line or add-on therapy. They are indicated in patients who suffer from asthma, diabetes, and peripheral vascular disease, as they do not adversely affect these conditions.

- **Angina** : Their vasodilating effect reduces workload on the heart.

ADRENERGIC BLOCKERS:

These drugs have been discussed in detail in Unit III. Both α and β blockers are used in the management of hypertension

β blockers:

- They act in two ways to reduce blood pressure. Firstly, they act directly on the heart to reduce cardiac output. Secondly, they reduce sympathetic stimulation to the kidney, which inhibits the release of renin.

- Selective β1 blockers, including metoprolol and atenolol are commonly prescribed. Non-selective blockers must be avoided in asthmatics, as they can cause bronchoconstriction.

- Adverse effects include bradycardia, hypotension, fatigue, and lethargy. Abrupt withdrawal of these drugs can induce angina or myocardial infarction. If discontinued, these drugs must always be tapered off.

- They are useful for primary treatment of hypertension, especially in patients with concomitant heart disease.

α blockers:

- These include the drugs prazocin, terazocin, and doxazocin.

- They reduce blood pressure by relaxing the smooth muscles of the vascular walls, which lowers peripheral vascular resistance.

- Adverse effects include postural hypotension and tachycardia. Long-term use can lead to congestive heart failure due to sodium and water retention.

- They are not used for initial treatment owing to their adverse effects, and are reserved for refractory cases.

Combined α/β blockers:

- These include the drugs labetalol and carvedilol.
- They produce pharmacological effects of both α and β blockers, resulting in a profound fall in blood pressure.
- Labetalol is indicated during hypertension of pregnancy, and hypertensive emergencies. Carvedilol is generally not used as an anti-hypertensive agent.

CENTRALLY ACTING α2 AGONISTS

- These drugs decrease sympathetic outflow to the periphery, resulting in fall in blood pressure and bradycardia. The drugs in this category are discussed completely in Unit III.
- Clonidine is indicated in patients with renal disease as it does not compromise renal blood flow. Methyldopa is indicated for hypertension in pregnancy.

VASODILATORS

- These include the drugs hydralazine, dihydralazine, and minoxidil.
- As the name suggests, these drugs cause vasodilation by relaxing the smooth muscles in the walls of arteries and arterioles.
- These agents tend to cause reflex stimulation of the heart. This leads to tachycardia, increased myocardial contractility, and increased workload and oxygen consumption. This can predispose to angina and myocardial infarction.
- They also increase renin secretion, and can cause sodium and water retention.
- For these reasons, vasodilators are always combined with beta blockers and diuretics.
- Hydralazine is used to manage hypertension in pregnancy. Topical minoxidil is used to treat alopecia and male pattern baldness.

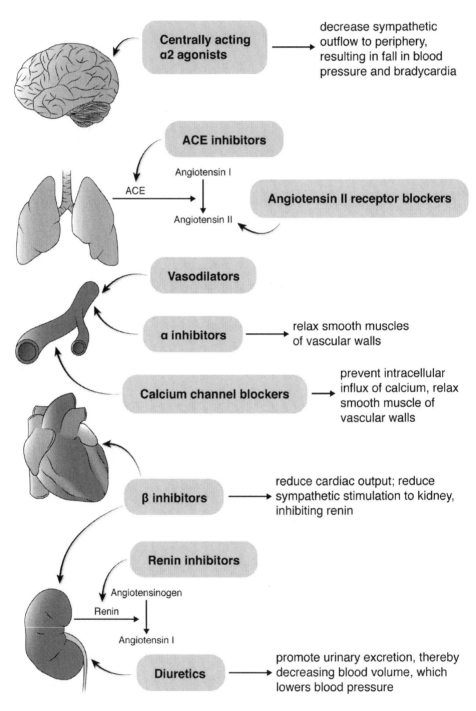

Centrally acting
α2 agonists → decrease sympathetic outflow to periphery, resulting in fall in blood pressure and bradycardia

ACE inhibitors

Angiotensin I

ACE

Angiotensin II

Angiotensin II receptor blockers

Vasodilators

α inhibitors → relax smooth muscles of vascular walls

Calcium channel blockers → prevent intracellular influx of calcium, relax smooth muscle of vascular walls

β inhibitors → reduce cardiac output; reduce sympathetic stimulation to kidney, inhibiting renin

Renin inhibitors

Angiotensinogen

Renin

Angiotensin I

Diuretics → promote urinary excretion, thereby decreasing blood volume, which lowers blood pressure

EXERCISES

1. Hypertension is a risk factor for development of all of the following diseases except:
   a. Heart disease
   b. Diabetes
   c. Stroke
   d. Kidney failure

2. Which of the following diuretics does not cause hypokalemia?
   a. Furosemide
   b. Hydrochlorothiazide
   c. Spironolactone
   d. Bumetanide

3. ACE inhibitors decrease the levels of which of the following?
   a. Renin
   b. Angiotensin I
   c. Angiotensin II
   d. None of the above

4. Which of the following ACE inhibitors has the longest plasma half-life?
   a. Captopril
   b. Lisinopril
   c. Enalapril
   d. Ramipril

5. Which of the following is not indicated as a primary drug for hypertension?
   a. Losartan
   b. Metoprolol
   c. Prazosin
   d. Chlorthalidone

6. Which of the following antihypertensives does not work on the renin-angiotensin system?
   a. Lisinopril
   b. Candesartan
   c. Atenolol
   d. Alisartan

7. Which of the following drugs can cause gingival hyperplasia?
   a. Verapamil
   b. Nifedipine
   c. Diltiazem
   d. Enalapril

8. Which of the following antihypertensives can cause AV heart block?
   a. Verapamil
   b. Nifedipine
   c. Diltiazem
   d. Enalapril

9. Which of the following anti-hypertensives is preferred for patients with renal disease?
   a. Minoxidil
   b. Methyldopa
   c. Clonidine
   d. Hydralazine

10. Which of the following drugs is indicated in male pattern baldness?
    a. Minoxidil
    b. Methyldopa
    c. Clonidine
    d. Hydralazine

CHAPTER 2

Drugs Used for Myocardial Ischemia

Myocardial ischemia is a condition of reduced blood flow to the myocardium. Blood to the heart usually comes from coronary arteries, so if there is a reduction in the diameter of these arteries, the blood flow can be compromised. The most common cause is atherosclerotic disease, where there is deposition of plaque on the walls of the coronary arteries. Uncommonly, other causes, such as vascular smooth muscle spasm, can also lead to myocardial ischemia.

Myocardial ischemia can lead to angina, or myocardial infarction. There are three types of angina – stable, unstable, and variant (or Prinzmetal) angina.

The drugs that are commonly used in the management of angina are summarized in Table 1.

Table 1. Drugs used in the management of angina

DRUG CATEGORY	EXAMPLE	PURPOSE
Nitrates	Glyceryl trinitrate, isosorbide dinitrate	To abort an established attack
Beta blockers	Propranolol, metoprolol, atenolol	Prophylaxis
Calcium channel blockers	Verapamil, diltiazem, nifedipine	Prophylaxis
Potassium channel openers	Nicorandil	Prophylaxis
Miscellaneous drugs	Ranolazine, trimetazidine	Prophylaxis

NITRATES

These are the first-line drugs used for relief from angina. Based on their onset and duration of action, they are classified as:

- Short-acting: e.g., Glyceryl trinitrate or nitroglycerin
- Long-acting: e.g., Isosorbide dinitrate

Mechanism of action:

- Organic nitrates are converted into nitrates, which in turn is converted into nitric oxide (NO).
- NO is a powerful vasodilator and acts by increasing the levels of cyclic GMP within cells.
- Elevated cGMP causes dephosphorylation of the myosin light chain, which causes relaxation of smooth muscles in the blood vessel walls.

Clinical actions:

Nitrates basically reduce the demand for oxygen from the myocardium. It does this by the following methods:

- **Reducing the preload** : Nitrates cause venous dilation, which decreases venous return to the heart and workload of the heart.
- **Reducing the afterload** : There is also arteriolar dilation, which decreases the peripheral resistance and afterload.
- **Improved coronary blood flow** : Direct dilation of coronary vasculature improves blood flow to the ischemic regions of the myocardium.
- **Other systemic effects** : Cutaneous vasodilation can cause flushing of skin. Bronchi and esophageal smooth muscles are relaxed slightly. There is decreased renal and splanchnic blood flow to compensate for the vasodilation in other areas.

Pharmacokinetics:

Nitroglycerin has high first-pass metabolism and is therefore not administered orally. The most preferred route is sublingual, from which it is quickly absorbed and acts within one minute. Longer acting drugs have better oral bioavailability, and their onset of action may take up to 30 minutes.

Adverse effects:

- Most common is headache due to vasodilation.
- Other effects include hypotension, tachycardia, and facial flushing.

Indications:

- **Angina** : Including stable, unstable, and variant angina. Short-acting nitrates are used to obtain immediate relief, while long-acting nitrates are used to reduce the frequency of anginal attacks.

- **Myocardial infarction and acute coronary syndromes** : It improves outcomes in these patients.

- **Esophageal spasm and achalasia** : Relieves spasm and promotes swallowing of food.

BETA BLOCKERS

- Beta adrenergic blockers block the β1 receptors of the heart. This decreases the heart rate, force of contraction, and cardiac output. All this serves to reduce the workload and oxygen demand of the myocardium.

- In patients with angina, they have the following therapeutic effects:

    o They decrease the frequency and severity of anginal attacks.
    o In stable angina, they improve exercise tolerance.
    o They improve mortality rates in patients who have had MI before, or who have cardiac failure.
    o Non-selective beta blockers must be avoided in patients with asthma.

CALCIUM CHANNEL BLOCKERS

- Calcium channel blockers cause vascular smooth muscle relaxation. Their main effect is on the coronary vessels. They also reduce the afterload on the heart by vasodilation of arterioles.

- They are used as prophylaxis in all three forms of angina. However, they are not recommended for use in myocardial infarction.

POTASSIUM CHANNEL OPENERS

- Nicorandil causes an influx of potassium into the cells. This causes hyperpolarization of vascular smooth muscle, resulting in vasodilation.

- There is arterial and venous dilation, as well as increase in coronary blood flow.

- It decreases the frequency of anginal attacks and improves exercise tolerance. It is also believed to have a 'cardioprotective effect' which prevents vascular occlusion.

- Adverse effects include headache, flushing, dizziness, nausea, and vomiting

MISCELLANEOUS DRUGS

Ranolazine:

- This drug is a sodium channel blocker. It prevents intracellular entry of sodium, which indirectly prevents calcium entry into cells. It thus functions similar to CCBs.
- It is reserved for patients in whom traditional antianginal therapy does not work.
- This drug can be administered orally. It has a bioavailability of 30 to 50%, and the onset of action takes 4 to 6 hours. It is metabolized in the liver, through the cytochrome P450 system, and is excreted out through the urine. The elimination half-life is about 7 hours.

Trimetazidine:

- The exact mechanism of action of this drug is uncertain, but it acts by non-hemodynamic mechanisms.
- It is useful in patients who are not responding to long-acting nitrates and CCBs.

PHARMACOTHERAPY IN MYOCARDIAL INFARCTION

Myocardial infarction (MI), or heart attack, is a condition where there is irreversible necrosis (infarction) of the cardiac muscle. This occurs secondary to prolonged ischemia. Once MI occurs, the goals of drug therapy are:

- To manage the patient's pain and anxiety
- To limit the spread and extent of the infarct
- To reduce the workload on the heart
- To reverse the cause. For instance, a blocked coronary artery must be recannulated to restore circulation to the myocardium

Prehospital care:

Along with providing supplemental oxygen, the following drugs are indicated:

- **Non-enteric coated aspirin** : This has antiplatelet actions that prevent initiation of blood clotting and help limit the infarct size.
- **Nitroglycerin** : This improves oxygen supply to the myocardium, and provides symptomatic relief from pain. However, it does not improve mortality rates.

In-hospital care:

- **Antithrombotic drugs** : This includes heparin and related drugs. These potentiate the action of anti-platelet drugs and prevent the formation of thrombi associated with MI.

- **Beta blockers** : These drugs reduce the workload of the heart and reduce its oxygen demand. They also have antiarrhythmic properties, and prevent ventricular ectopy following MI.

- **ACE inhibitors or angiotensin receptor blockers** : They also reduce cardiac workload, especially in patients with ventricular dysfunction.

- **Thrombolytic drugs** : These are meant to dissolve the blood clot in the occluded vessels and restore circulation. Fibrinolytic drugs, including streptokinase, urokinase, and alteplase are used for this purpose.

- **Analgesics** : During this episode, it is essential to ensure that the patient has relief from pain and anxiety. Morphine sulphate is the drug of choice.

EXERCISES

1. Which of the following drugs is used to abort an established anginal attack?
   a. Glyceryl trinitrate
   b. Isosorbide dinitrate
   c. Propranolol
   d. Verapamil

2. Which of the following compounds is increased within the cell by the action of nitrates?
   a. ATP
   b. cAMP
   c. GTP
   d. cGMP

3. What is the most common side effect of nitrate drugs?
   a. Headache
   b. Nausea and vomiting
   c. Renal dysfunction
   d. Tachycardia

4. Which of the following drugs has a cardioprotective effect on the heart?
   a. Atenolol
   b. Nicorandil
   c. Isosorbide dinitrate
   d. Diltiazem

5. Which of the following anti-anginal drugs does not have a hemodynamic mechanism of action?
   a. Verapamil
   b. Metoprolol
   c. Trimetazidine
   d. Nicorandil

6. Which of the following drugs must not be used for angina patients who have asthma?

a. Verapamil
b. Propranolol
c. Trimetazidine
d. Nicorandil

7. What is the bioavailability of ranolazine?
   a. 10-20%
   b. 20-40%
   c. 30-50%
   d. 50-70%

8. Which is the analgesic drug of choice during a myocardial infarction?
   a. Codeine
   b. Tramadol
   c. Morphine
   d. Ketorolac

9. Which of the following drugs does not improve mortality rates after myocardial infarction?
   a. Propranolol
   b. Aspirin
   c. Nitroglycerin
   d. Enalapril

10. Which of the following drugs is used to lyse the blood clot after an MI?
    a. Aspirin
    b. Alteplase
    c. Atenolol
    d. Heparin

CHAPTER 3

Drugs Used in Arrhythmias

The cardiac muscle is specialized in that it does not require external stimulus to facilitate contraction. The heart contains a special group of 'pacemaker' cells that automatically generate action potentials in a rhythmic fashion. Any defect in the generation or conduction of this action potential can result in arrhythmias. The different kinds of arrhythmias that can commonly occur are summarized in Table 1.

Table 1. Types of arrhythmias

CATEGORY OF ARRHYTHMIA	TYPES
Atrial Arrhythmias	Atrial flutter
	Atrial fibrillation
Supraventricular tachycardias	AV nodal entry
	Acute supraventricular tachycardia
	Paroxysmal supraventricular tachycardia
Ventricular tachycardias	Acute ventricular tachycardia
	Ventricular fibrillation
	Torsades de pointes
Disorders of conduction	A-V block: first, second, and third degree block

Antiarrhythmic drugs prevent arrhythmias by modifying impulse generation or impulse conduction, or they reduce symptoms associated with arrhythmias. To achieve this, these drugs must act at some phase of the action potential. Antiarrhythmic drugs may be classified based on the specific phase of the action potential at which they act. This is summarized in Table 2.

Table 2. Classification of Antiarrhythmic Drugs

DRUG CLASS	PHASE OF ACTION POTENTIAL BLOCKED	DRUG CATEGORY	EXAMPLES
Class IA	Phase 0 depolarization in ventricular muscle fibers- slows	Sodium channel blockers	Quinidine, procainamide
Class IB	Phase 3 repolarization in ventricular muscle fibers - shortens		Lidocaine, mexiletine
Class IC	Phase 0 depolarization in ventricular muscle fibers- greatly slows		Flecainide, propafenone
Class II	Phase IV depolarization in SA and AV nodes	β adrenergic blocker	Metoprolol, esmolol
Class III	Phase 3 repolarization in ventricular muscle fibers - prolongs	Potassium channel blocker	Amiodarone, dronedarone
Class IV	Inhibits action potential generation in SA and AV nodes	Calcium channel blocker	Verapamil, diltiazem

CLASS I ANTIARRHYTHMIC DRUGS

These are sodium channel blockers. They prevent sodium ions from entering the cell, thereby preventing depolarization.

CLASS IA DRUGS

They bind to open and inactivated sodium channels, and act during phase 0 of depolarization.

Quinidine:

- This drug also blocks α-adrenergic receptors and cholinergic receptors. Other class I drugs do not possess this activity.
- It is rapidly absorbed after oral administration. It is metabolized by the cytochrome P450 system. Metabolites are active.
- **Adverse effects**: Blurred vision, tinnitus, headache, disorientation, and psychosis. There is also a high risk of cardiac arrest, and other arrhythmias like torsades de pointes.

- **Indications**: Quinidine may be used for all types of arrhythmias such as atrial, AV-junctional, and ventricular tachyarrhythmias.

Procainamide:

- Procainamide is used to treat acute atrial and ventricular arrhythmias.
- It is short-acting and the effect lasts for about 2 to 3 hours.

Disopyramide:

- It has cardiac depressant effects, and mild anticholinergic actions.
- Disopyramide is used in atrial fibrillation and flutter, to maintain normal sinus rhythm.
- It is well absorbed orally. About 50% of the drug is metabolized in the liver through the cytochrome P450 system and the rest is excreted unchanged in urine.
- Anticholinergic adverse effects: Dry mouth, blurred vision, constipation, and urinary retention.

CLASS IB ANTIARRHYTHMIC DRUGS:

These drugs rapidly bind to and rapidly dissociate from the sodium channels. They tend to function when the channels are in an inactivated state, and are useful when the heart 'fires' rapidly.

Lignocaine:

- Primarily a local anesthetic, it suppresses spontaneous firing from ectopic foci.
- It is commonly employed in ventricular fibrillation and pulseless ventricular tachycardia.
- It is given intravenously to avoid high first-pass metabolism. The other details of this drug are discussed in Unit IV.

Mexiletine:

- This drug is pharmacologically similar to lignocaine and functions in a similar manner.
- It is completely absorbed through the oral route, metabolized in the liver, and excreted through urine. The plasma half-life is about 9 to 12 hours.
- It is indicated for chronic treatment of ventricular arrhythmias.

CLASS IC ANTIARRHYTHMIC DRUGS

This is the most potent category in this class. They act on sodium channels in the open state and markedly delay conduction.

Propafenone:

- Slows conduction in all cardiac pathways. In addition, it has some β-blocking action.
- **Adverse effects**: Bitter taste, nausea, vomiting, blurred vision, constipation.
- It is indicated for atrial arrhythmias and paroxysmal supraventricular tachycardias.

Flecainide:

- This drug also blocks potassium channels, which further prolongs the action potential.
- It is absorbed orally, metabolized in the liver by cytochrome P450 system, and excreted in urine.
- It can cause dizziness, nausea, and blurred vision. It may aggravate chronic heart failure due to its negative inotropic effect.
- It is indicated in resistant cases of atrial fibrillation, and life-threatening ventricular tachycardia in patients who do not have congestive cardiac failure.

CLASS II ANTIARRHYTHMIC DRUGS

- These are beta blockers, which work by suppressing sympathetic activity.
- They slow the phase 4 of depolarization, which helps to prolong AV conduction, and decreases the heart rate and force of contraction.
- Metoprolol is most commonly used. Esmolol, which is short-acting, is preferred for acute arrhythmias that require immediate management.
- The main antiarrhythmic indications of beta blockers are:
  o Atrial flutter and atrial fibrillation
  o AV nodal reentrant tachycardia
  o Following MI, they prevent ventricular arrhythmias, which can be fatal.

CLASS III ANTIARRHYTHMIC DRUGS

These are potassium channel blockers. They prevent the outflow of potassium from the cells during the repolarization phase. Thus, they prolong the refractory period that immediately follows the action potential.

AMIODARONE:

Amiodarone and dronedarone are potassium channel blockers that exhibit some degree of Class I, II, and IV activity as well. They also block α-adrenergic receptors to some extent.

Pharmacokinetics:

On oral administration, the drug is absorbed slowly and incompletely. Therefore, onset of action may take days to weeks. Intravenous injection of the drug can produce rapid onset. It is stored in adipose tissue and skeletal muscle, from where it is slowly released. The plasma half-life is 3 to 8 weeks. Metabolism occurs in the liver, through the cytochrome P450 system.

Adverse effects:

- Corneal deposits, optic neuritis, bluish-grey discoloration of skin.
- Nausea, vomiting, hepatotoxicity
- Can cause hypothyroidism or hyperthyroidism.
- Prolonged use may cause pulmonary alveolitis and fibrosis.

Indications:

- Drug of choice for atrial fibrillation and flutter
- Supraventricular tachycardias, ventricular tachyarrhythmias.

SOTALOL:

- This is a Class III agent that also has properties of non-selective β blockers.
- It is preferred for patients with left ventricular hypertrophy or atherosclerotic heart disease. In these patients, it is indicated for atrial fibrillation, atrial flutter, or supraventricular tachycardia.

CLASS IV ANTIARRHYTHMIC DRUGS

- These are calcium channel blockers and include the drugs verapamil and diltiazem.
- These drugs bind selectively to the open, depolarized, voltage-sensitive calcium channels, and prevent inward movement of calcium. This prevents repolarization from occurring until the drug dissociates from the channel.
- The SA nodes and AV nodes are dependent on calcium to generate current, and these drugs can inhibit this process.
- They reduce ventricular rate in atrial flutter and fibrillation. They are also used for the management of supraventricular tachycardia.

OTHER DRUGS USED IN ARRHYTHMIA

Adenosine:

- This is a naturally occurring nucleoside, which forms an important component of DNA, RNA, and energy compounds.

- At high doses, it can inhibit automatic firing of the AV node, can decrease conduction velocity, and can prolong the refractory period.
- It has a short onset of action (10 to 15 seconds) and is ideal for use in acute supraventricular tachycardia.
- **Adverse effects**: Hypotension, chest pain, flushing.

MAGNESIUM SULFATE:

- Magnesium is a dietary mineral. In the body, one of its main functions is to facilitate transport of ions such as sodium, potassium, and calcium across cell membranes.
- When administered intravenously, it can retard impulse generation from the SA node. It can also prolong conduction.
- It is indicated for life threatening arrhythmias, including digoxin-induced arrhythmias and torsades de pointes.

EXERCISES
---

1. Which class of antiarrhythmic drugs does lignocaine belong to?
   a. Class IA
   b. Class IB
   c. Class II
   d. Class IC

2. Which ion channel is blocked by Class I antiarrhythmic agents?
   a. Sodium
   b. Potassium
   c. Calcium
   d. Chloride

3. Which of the following drugs had anticholinergic effects?
   a. Quinidine
   b. Procainamide
   c. Disopyramide
   d. Lignocaine

4. What is the plasma half-life of mexiletine?
   a. 2 to 3 hours
   b. 4 to 5 hours
   c. 7 to 8 hours
   d. 9 to 12 hours

5. Which of the following drugs has potassium channel blocking, as well as β blocking effects?
   a. Atenolol
   b. Propranolol
   c. Sotalol
   d. Esmolol

6. Which of the following drugs can cause pulmonary fibrosis?
   a. Quinidine
   b. Sotalol
   c. Amiodarone
   d. Magnesium sulfate

7. What is the drug of choice for atrial fibrillation and flutter?
   a. Digoxin
   b. Amiodarone
   c. Metoprolol
   d. Adenosine

8. What is the mechanism of action of potassium channel blockers?
   a. Prevent generation of impulse
   b. Retard depolarization
   c. Prolong refractory period
   d. Inhibit impulse conduction

9. Which nucleoside is used as an antiarrhythmic agent?
   a. Guanosine
   b. Adenosine
   c. Thymidine
   d. Inosine

10. When used for management of arrhythmias, what route must magnesium sulfate be administered?
    a. Oral
    b. Sublingual
    c. Intramuscular
    d. Intravenous

CHAPTER 4

Drugs Used in Heart Failure

Heart failure is a condition where the heart fails to pump enough blood to meet the needs of the body. While the body initially tries to compensate, ultimately, a lot of pathological changes occur in the heart. A short summary of pathological changes that occur in heart failure is given below:

- Initially, low cardiac output results in a drop in blood pressure. This is detected by the baroreceptors, which in turn cause sympathetic stimulation.
- Sympathetic activity stimulates the beta-adrenergic receptors. This increases the force of contraction of the heart. However, β stimulation also causes vasoconstriction. This increases venous return, and the pre-load. The workload of the heart increases.
- Low cardiac output also decreases renal perfusion, which stimulates renin release. The renin-angiotensin-aldosterone system causes sodium and water retention, increasing the blood volume. This further increases cardiac workload.
- To compensate for the excess workload, there is hypertrophy of cardiac muscle. While initially this may increase the force of contraction, ultimately the fibers elongate, weaken, and the force of contraction lessens.
- Therefore, although the heart can initially compensate, over time, there is decompensated heart failure. In decompensated heart failure, there is edema due to fluid retention, dyspnea, and fatigue.

AIMS OF THERAPY IN HEART FAILURE

The therapeutic aims in heart failure are as follows:

- Improve inotropic effect on the heart, without increasing the workload
- Decrease fluid retention and promote excretion of sodium and water
- Inhibition of the sympathetic nervous system

DRUGS THAT IMPROVE FORCE OF CONTRACTION:

Certain drugs are used to improve the force of contraction of the heart, which in turn improves the cardiac output. These are referred to as inotropic drugs.

CARDIAC GLYCOSIDES

Cardiac glycosides are drugs that increase the inotropic activity of the heart by influencing the flow of sodium and calcium ions. They come from the foxglove plant and are collectively referred to as digitalis. The main cardiac glycoside in use today is digoxin.

Mechanism of action:

- This drug inhibits the enzyme Na+/K+ ATPase, which is responsible for pumping sodium out of the cell.
- The increased intracellular sodium increases the concentration gradient, which stimulates the Na+/Ca2+ exchanger pump. This drives calcium into the cell. The increased calcium is available for the next excitation-contraction coupling, and increases the force of contraction

Clinical actions:

- **Heart** : It has the following effects
  o **Positive inotropic effect**: increases force of contraction of the heart. It shortens systole and prolongs diastole.
  o Decreases heart rate, causing bradycardia
  o Depresses generation and conduction of the action potential

- **Kidney** : Causes diuresis due to increased circulation and renal perfusion
- **CNS** : Stimulates chemoreceptor trigger zone, leading to nausea and vomiting. Can cause some amount of mental confusion, disorientation, and visual disturbances.

Pharmacokinetics:

It is available in both oral and intravenous forms. On oral administration, bioavailability is about 60-80%. After absorption, 25% of it is bound to plasma proteins, and the rest is widely distributed. It gets concentrated in the heart, skeletal muscle, liver, and kidney.

The onset of action occurs in 15 to 30 minutes. It does not undergo metabolism, and is excreted unchanged in the urine. Plasma half-life is about 40 hours.

Adverse effects:

- Blurred or yellowish vision
- Anorexia, nausea, and vomiting
- Can induce different kinds of arrhythmias.

Indications:

- Congestive cardiac failure
- **Cardiac arrhythmias**: Including atrial fibrillation, and paroxysmal supraventricular tachycardias.

BETA-ADRENERGIC AGONISTS

- The commonly used inotropic drugs in this category are dobutamine and dopamine.
- These drugs increase cyclic AMP levels, which activate protein kinase. This in turn causes phosphorylation of slow calcium channels, and increases calcium entry into the myocardial cells, this enhances muscle contraction.
- They are used intravenously for management of acute heart failure in the hospital setting, and cannot be used for long-term.

DRUGS THAT DECREASE FLUID RETENTION

ANGIOTENSIN-CONVERTING ENZYME (ACE) INHIBITORS:

- These drugs inhibit angiotensin II and aldosterone. This prevents sodium and water retention. They also cause vasodilation. Both these effects reduce the preload and afterload on the heart.
- They are indicated in all stages of left ventricular failure, and in heart failure with reduced ejection fraction.
- ACE inhibitors increase bradykinin levels, and may predispose to angioedema. In patients who cannot tolerate them, angiotensin-receptor blockers may be used instead.

DIURETICS:

- Diuretics promote excretion of sodium and water by the kidneys. This relieves the congestion and edema that occurs in heart failure.
- Loop diuretics such as furosemide are the most effective diuretics. Thiazide diuretics are not useful.
- They promptly relieve symptoms of heart failure, such as dyspnea and orthopnea. However, they do not improve mortality rate, and must be used with other agents such as beta blockers or ACE inhibitors.

DRUGS THAT INHIBIT THE SYMPATHETIC NERVOUS SYSTEM

- Beta adrenergic blockers are the main class of drugs that are used to suppress the sympathetic overactivity that occurs in heart failure.
- Beta-blockers are actually known for their negative inotropic effect. However, they do have more benefit in patients with heart failure, as they reduce the oxygen demand and consumption by the myocardium.
- These drugs also inhibit release of renin from the kidneys.

EXERCISES

1. Which of the following is not a primary management goal in heart failure?
   a. Decrease fluid retention
   b. Inhibit sympathetic activity
   c. Inhibit electrical activity
   d. Improve force of contraction

2. Which enzyme is inhibited by digoxin?
   a. Kinase
   b. Na+/K+ ATPase
   c. Angiotensin converting enzyme
   d. Phosphorylase

3. Which of the following ions promotes cardiac muscle contraction?
   a. Sodium
   b. Calcium
   c. Potassium
   d. Chloride

4. What is the bioavailability of digoxin when administered by oral route?
   a. 10-20%
   b. 20-40%
   c. 40-60%
   d. 60-80%

5. What is the time of onset of action of digoxin?
   a. 10-15 minutes
   b. 15-30 minutes
   c. 30-45 minutes
   d. 45-60 minutes

6. Which drug is preferred for the management of acute heart failure in the hospital setting?
   a. Adrenaline
   b. Dopamine
   c. Digoxin
   d. Adenosine

7. What compound is increased by beta adrenergic agonists?
   a. ATP
   b. cAMP
   c. GTP
   d. cGMP

8. Which of the following classes of diuretics is preferred for symptomatic relief in heart failure?
   a. Loop diuretics
   b. Thiazide diuretics
   c. Osmotic diuretics
   d. Potassium sparing diuretics

9. Which of the following drugs does not improve mortality rates in heart failure?
   a. Metoprolol
   b. Digoxin
   c. Enalapril
   d. Furosemide

10. What is the reason for using beta-blockers in heart failure?
    a. Negative inotropic effect
    b. Vasodilation
    c. Inhibition of sympathetic activity
    d. Bradycardia effect

UNIT VII : HEMATOPOIETIC SYSTEM

Hematinics and Drugs Affecting Blood Clotting

The hematopoietic system consists of the red blood cells, white blood cells, and platelets. The most common diseases that affect this system are anemia, thrombotic diseases, and bleeding disorders.

DRUGS USED TO TREAT ANEMIAS

Anemia is a condition where there is a decrease in concentration of circulating plasma hemoglobin. It occurs due to a wide variety of causes. Broadly, anemia may be genetic or acquired. Acquired anemia can be due to nutritional deficiencies, chronic blood loss, infections, and other conditions. Accordingly, a wide variety of drugs are available to treat anemia, which are described in this chapter.

Iron:

- The heme component of hemoglobin consists of four molecules of iron. Apart from this, iron is also combined with storage proteins (as ferritin), or with transport proteins (as transferrin). Iron is largely obtained from the diet. If nutritional intake is not adequate, or if there is excessive blood loss, iron deficiency anemia may occur. This may be corrected by taking supplements of elemental iron.

- **Pharmacokinetics**: Iron is usually absorbed from the intestine in the ferrous form. Hence it is administered orally as ferrous sulphate, ferrous gluconate, or ferrous aluminum citrate. Parenteral preparations are also available as iron dextran or iron sucrose.

- **Adverse effects:** Abdominal pain, constipation, diarrhea, and black stools can occur with oral administration. Parenteral administration can cause anaphylaxis.

Folic acid:

- Like iron, this is primarily used to address deficiency states. This can occur during pregnancy, alcoholism, small intestine diseases, or during therapy with certain drugs that inhibit the enzyme dihydrofolate reductase (e.g. Methotrexate).

- It is indicated for treatment and prophylaxis against megaloblastic anemia, caused due to folate deficiency.
- It is absorbed from intestinal jejunum, and excess is excreted unchanged. No side effects are reported.

Cyanocobalamin:

- This is vitamin B12. It is deficient in pernicious anemia, a condition where the gastric parietal cells fail to produce the 'intrinsic factor' required for its absorption. Dietary deficiency may also occur, and megaloblastic anemia may require combination treatment with vitamin B12 and folate. Other conditions, like malabsorption syndromes and gastric resection may contribute to deficiency.
- It is administered parenterally in pernicious anemia. For other types of deficiency, it may be administered orally along with folate. It does not have adverse effects.

Erythropoietin:

- This is a glycoprotein that is synthesized in the kidney. It stimulates differentiation of proerythroblasts and release of reticulocytes into the bloodstream.
- Human erythropoietin, called epoetin alfa, produced by recombinant DNA technology, is indicated for anemia secondary to bone marrow disorders and end-stage renal disease.
- Adverse effects usually occur due to sudden increase in hematocrit. This increases risk of clot formation, especially around the A-V shunts in patients on dialysis.

Hydroxyurea:

- This is largely used in sickle cell anemia. It reduces the frequency of sickle crises.
- This increases the levels of fetal hemoglobin and dilutes the abnormal hemoglobin. However, it can cause bone marrow suppression and cutaneous vasculitis.
- It is also used in chronic myeloblastic anemia and polycythemia vera.

Pentoxifylline:

- This drug improves the flexibility of erythrocytes and reduces blood viscosity.
- Its clinical effects are to improve blood flow, enhance tissue oxygenation, and reduce systemic vascular resistance.
- It is indicated in conditions where there is reduced blood flow to the tissues, such as intermittent claudication, diabetic angiopathies, osteoradionecrosis, and leg ulcers.

DRUGS AFFECTING BLOOD COAGULATION

Blood coagulation is a normal physiological response to insult or injury. While this is beneficial after injury, sometimes intrinsic coagulation can cause thrombus formation which can lead to ischemic conditions. There are two phases of blood coagulation - the initial phase in which platelet aggregation occurs, and the final phase marked by the coagulation cascade. Drugs are categorized based on the phase on which they act.

ANTIPLATELET DRUGS

These drugs inhibit the formation of the initial blood clot, or the platelet plug.

Aspirin:

- Aspirin inactivates the cyclo-oxygenase enzyme-1, which in turn inhibits the formation of thromboxane A2 which is responsible for platelet aggregation. Thus, aspirin inhibits platelet aggregation.

- For antiplatelet action, the recommended dose is around 75mg a day. It is well absorbed from the oral route, and is converted to salicylic acid in the liver. The half-life of salicylic acid lasts up to 12 hours, after which it is metabolized and excreted in the urine.

- Aspirin prolongs bleeding time. It can also cause occult GI bleeds.

Ticlopidine, clopidogrel, and prasugrel:

- These compounds prevent binding of ATP to platelet surface receptors, thereby inhibiting platelet aggregation.

- These agents can be taken orally. Food interferes with absorption of only ticlopidine. After absorption, these drugs bind to plasma proteins, and are metabolized in the liver. Excretion occurs through urine and feces.

- Ticlopidine can cause serious adverse reactions such as agranulocytosis, aplastic anemia, and purpura. All these drugs can cause prolonged bleeding.

Glycoprotein receptor antagonists:

- Drugs such as abciximab, eptifibatide, and tirofiban act by inhibiting glycoprotein IIb/IIIa receptors, which usually facilitates binding of fibrinogen and von Willebrand factor, and leads to platelet aggregation.

- These drugs are usually given intravenously, and act within 30 minutes. They are rapidly cleared from plasma and excreted in urine. However, the antiplatelet effect of a single dose can act up to 48 hours.

Dipyridamole:

- This drug inhibits the enzyme cyclic nucleotide phosphodiesterase. This reduces intracellular cAMP levels and suppresses thromboxane A2 formation.

- It is used from oral route, is highly bound to plasma proteins, undergoes glucuronide conjugation in the liver, and is excreted in feces.
- It can cause vasodilation and is contraindicated in patients with unstable angina, as this can get worsened.

Indications of antiplatelet drugs:
- Patients with evidence of coronary artery disease
- Acute coronary syndromes, including unstable angina and myocardial infarction
- Cerebrovascular disease
- Patients with prosthetic heart valves and AV shunts
- Venous thromboembolism, for prophylaxis and treatment

ANTITHROMBOTIC DRUGS:
These drugs inhibit the coagulation cascade, or the formation of the final blood clot.

Heparin and heparin analogues:
- Heparin is an anticoagulant that occurs naturally in the body in the lungs, liver, and intestinal mucosa. It is present along with histamine in the mast cells. For pharmacotherapy, heparin derived from porcine sources are produced in two forms:
  o Unfractionated heparin (UFH)
  o Low-molecular-weight heparins (LMWH) – enoxaparin, dalteparin, and tinzaparin
- Mechanism of action: Heparin binds with antithrombin III, and this complex inactivates factors II and X of the clotting cascade.
- Pharmacokinetics: UFH is administered intravenously, while LMWH may be administered subcutaneously. It binds to several proteins and is metabolized by the monocyte macrophage system. Metabolites are excreted in urine.
- Adverse effects:
  o Excessive bleeding. This may be reversed by using the antidote protamine sulfate.
  o Allergic reactions, including anaphylaxis
  o Thrombocytopenia
- Indications: Prevention and management of venous thromboembolism.

Synthetic anticoagulants:
- Fondaparinux binds to antithrombin III and selectively inhibits factor Xa.
- It is administered subcutaneously, and has a more predictable pharmacokinetic profile than heparin. It is eliminated unchanged in urine. Plasma t1/2 is 17 to 21 hours.

Directly acting oral anticoagulants:

- These are drugs which do not need to bind to antithrombin III, and instead, directly act to inactivate clotting factors. Dabigatran directly inhibits thrombin formation, while rivaroxaban and apixaban directly inhibit factor Xa.

- All these drugs are taken orally. Rivaroxaban and apixaban are highly bound to plasma proteins and are metabolized in the liver by the cytochrome P450 system. All these drugs are substrates for glycoprotein P, with which they bind before being eliminated through urine and feces.

- These drugs have the potential to cause severe bleeding, and unlike heparin, they do not have approved antidotes. Dabigatran is contraindicated in patients with prosthetic heart valves.

- These drugs are used for prophylaxis against venous thromboembolism, and against stroke in patients with atrial fibrillation.

Warfarin:

- This is the only clinically used coumarin anticoagulant; related compounds are used as pesticides.

- Warfarin and other coumarin compounds decrease the regeneration of vitamin K from vitamin K epoxide. This decreases available levels of vitamin K. Vitamin K activates clotting factors II, VII, IX, and X, and this process is inhibited when warfarin is administered.

- Warfarin may be taken orally. It binds to plasma albumin, and can cross the placenta but not other barriers. It is contraindicated in pregnancy. It is metabolized in the liver by cytochrome P450 system and glucuronide conjugation, and is excreted in the urine. Its half-life is 40 hours.

- Warfarin therapy requires frequent monitoring of International Normalized Ratio (INR), which must be maintained in the range of 2 to 3. It is primarily used for prevention of stroke and venous thromboembolism.

- The main adverse effect is hemorrhage. Mild bleeding may be reversed by administration of vitamin K, while major bleeding may require transfusion with whole blood, plasma, or plasma concentrate. Another adverse effect is 'purple toe syndrome' where there is discoloration of the toes due to cholesterol plaque deposits.

Fibrinolytic drugs

- These are drugs that act to destroy existing blood clots. These agents promote the conversion of plasminogen to plasmin. Plasmin hydrolyzes fibrin and dissolves blood clots. The commonly used fibrinolytic drugs include streptokinase, urokinase, and alteplase.

- Fibrinolytic therapy is mainly used to lyse clots after myocardial infarction, to establish reperfusion. These drugs must be administered early, within 2-6 hours, as the clot becomes difficult to disintegrate as it ages. When the clot is broken down, the small fragments may stimulate platelet aggregation and further thrombosis. To prevent this, it is best to use these drugs along with antiplatelet and antithrombotic drugs.

- Alteplase is a 'fibrin selective' drug and acts locally at the site of blood clots. It binds only to plasminogen in blood clots, but not to tissue plasminogen.

DRUGS USED FOR BLEEDING TENDENCIES

Vitamin K

- This is a fat-soluble vitamin. Its main site of action is in the liver, where it acts as a cofactor for synthesis of four clotting factors – II, VII, IX, and X. Any deficiency of vitamin K can lead to bleeding tendencies. This may manifest as GI bleeds, hematuria, nasal bleeds, and skin ecchymosis.
- Vitamin K therapy is indicated in the following cases:
  o True deficiency due to poor diet, prolonged antimicrobial therapy, and malabsorption syndromes
  o Liver diseases
  o Deficiency in the newborn child
  o Overdose of oral anticoagulants such as warfarin
- Local hemostatic agents
- Hemostatic agents, or styptics are drugs that act locally at the site of injury to stop bleeding. These substances work by different mechanisms.
- Gelatin foam, oxidized cellulose, and fibrin usually provide a mesh framework for the clot to form. Thrombin powder directly stimulates clot formation, and is useful in patients with bleeding disorders.
- Vasoconstrictors such as adrenaline may also be applied locally. However, once the effect wears off, there may be reactionary bleeding.

Anti-fibrinolytic drugs

- Contrary to fibrinolytics, these drugs inhibit the conversion of plasminogen into plasmin. They usually bind to the lysine binding site on plasminogen and prevent its conversion.
- Aminocaproic acid and tranexamic acid are two commonly used antifibrinolytics. Tranexamic acid is 7-10 times more potent than aminocaproic acid. Both are administered via the oral route, and are excreted in urine. They can also be used topically for control of bleeding.
- It is used to control bleeding in patients with bleeding disorders, following trauma or minor procedures such as tooth extraction.

EXERCISES

1. Which of the following forms of anemia requires parenteral therapy?
   a. Microcytic anemia
   b. Megaloblastic anemia
   c. Pernicious anemia
   d. Sickle cell anemia

2. Which of the following drugs is preferred in sickle cell anemia?
   a. Iron
   b. Cyanocobalamin
   c. Erythropoietin
   d. Hydroxyurea

3. Which of the following drugs prevents binding of ATP to platelet receptors?
   a. Tirofiban
   b. Aspirin
   c. Clopidogrel
   d. Dipyridamole

4. What is the dose of aspirin for antiplatelet therapy?
   a. 50mg
   b. 75mg
   c. 100mg
   d. 325mg

5. What is the antidote for heparin-induced bleeding?
   a. Vitamin K
   b. Tranexemic acid
   c. Protamine sulfate
   d. Oxidised cellulose

6. Which of the following drugs selectively inhibits factor II?
   a. Enoxaparin
   b. Dabigatran
   c. Fondaparinux
   d. Rivaroxaban

7. What is the plasma half-life of warfarin?
   a. 10 hours
   b. 20 hours
   c. 30 hours
   d. 40 hours

8. What is the period within which fibrinolytic drugs must be administered after an MI?
   a. 2 hours
   b. 3 hours
   c. 5 hours
   d. 6 hours

9. Which of the following drugs inhibits the conversion of plasminogen into plasmin?
   a. Streptokinase
   b. Tranexemic acid
   c. Adrenaline
   d. Warfarin

10. Which of the following drugs acts 'locally' on the blood clot?
    a. Streptokinase
    b. Urokinase
    c. Alteplase
    d. Tranexemic acid

UNIT VIII : RESPIRATORY SYSTEM

Drugs Used in Cough and Bronchial Asthma

Respiratory disorders can involve the upper or lower respiratory tract. This chapter discusses two important conditions - cough and bronchial asthma.

DRUGS USED TO MANAGE COUGH

Cough is a defense mechanism of the respiratory tract against irritants. This is usually secondary to infection or allergy. Whenever possible, the underlying etiology of the cough must be ascertained and treated, along with treatment for cough itself. The following categories of drugs are used to manage cough.

Antitussives:

- Antitussives directly control the cough reflex mechanism by working at the central or peripheral part of the cough reflex arc.

- **Opioids**: These increase the stimulus threshold in the central cough center. Codeine and ethylmorphine are commonly used opioids. They have the potential for respiratory depression and must not be used in asthmatics. They can also cause constipation.

- **Non-opioids**: Dextromethorphan is a synthetic NMDA antagonist and works similar to opioids. It has a lower addictive profile, and does not cause respiratory depression.

- **Benzonatate**: This works peripherally to suppress the cough reflex receptors that are located in the lungs and respiratory passages. It may cause numbness of the tongue, mouth and throat, especially if the active drug comes in direct contact with the mucosa.

- **Indications for anti-tussives**: Dry, non-productive cough; especially cough that disturbs sleep, or may be detrimental to health (e.g. in patients with hernia, or who have had ocular surgery).

Pharyngeal demulcents:

- These are marketed as cough lozenges or syrups.

217

- They contain a combination of active ingredients, including honey, peppermint oil, anesthetics such as benzocaine, or dextromethorphan.
- They decrease afferent impulses sent from inflamed pharyngeal mucosa, by soothing the throat.

Expectorants:

- These drugs either increase bronchial secretions, or reduce their viscosity, thus facilitating their expulsion.
- Guaifenesin is a plant product which enhances mucociliary function and decreases the viscosity of secretions.
- Bromhexine is also a mucolytic and mucokinetic. It breaks down sputum by enhancing release of lysosomal enzymes and depolymerizing mucopolysaccharides. Adverse effects include nausea, gastric irritation, lacrimation, and rhinorrhea. Its metabolite, ambroxol, has similar effects.
- Carbocisteine and acetylcysteine: These drugs also liquify sputum, by breaking down disulphide bonds of proteins in mucous. However, it may also break down the gastric mucosal barrier, and must be avoided in patients prone to peptic ulcer.

DRUGS FOR BRONCHIAL ASTHMA

Asthma is a disease characterized by chronic inflammation of the bronchial airway, which leads to bronchoconstriction and increased bronchial secretions. Therapy is aimed at providing symptomatic relief, as well as reducing inflammation in the long-term.

Bronchodilators

- These drugs provide symptomatic relief by causing relaxation of the bronchial smooth muscles. The drugs used are β-2 agonists, methylxanthines, or anticholinergic drugs.

β-2 agonists:

These drugs directly act on the bronchial smooth muscle to relax it. There are two types of drugs used for asthma:

- Short acting β-2 agonists:
  - o These drugs are used for quick relief of acute bronchoconstriction. They do not have any anti-inflammatory effect, and must not be used as monotherapy in chronic asthma. They may be used alone only in intermittent asthma and in patients with exercise-induced bronchospasm.
  - o The onset of action is 15 to 30 minutes and the effects last for 4 to 6 hours.
  - o Drugs in this category include albuterol, levalbuterol, and terbutaline.

- Long acting β-2 agonists:
  o These drugs have a longer duration of action for at least 12 hours. As the onset is slow, they are not preferred for acute relief.
  o Salmeterol and formoterol are the drugs used in this category.
  o These drugs are not preferred as monotherapy. They may be used in combination with other drugs for management of moderate and severe persistent asthma.

Methylxanthines:

- Methylxanthines include the drugs caffeine, theophylline, and theobromine. Of these, theophylline has been used for the management of asthma and COPD.
- Theophylline causes bronchial smooth muscle relaxation. It also decreases the release of histamine from mast cells, and thereby exerts an anti-inflammatory effect.
- It has a narrow therapeutic window and several adverse effects. These include headache, nervousness, nausea, and gastric pain. Due to this, it is no longer considered as a first-line drug to treat asthma.

Anticholinergics:

- Anticholinergic drugs block M3 receptors which mediate bronchoconstriction.
- The commonly used drug is ipratropium bromide. It can be used for asthmatic exacerbations when short-acting β-2 agonists are not tolerable.
- Adverse effects include dry mouth and altered taste.

ANTI-INFLAMMATORY DRUGS

These drugs reduce the inflammation of the bronchial mucosa.

Corticosteroids:

- This is the drug of choice in all patients with persistent asthma, either with or without long-acting β-2 agonists. These drugs exert an anti-inflammatory effect by inhibiting the enzyme phospholipase-A2, which plays a key role in prostaglandin synthesis.
- Usually, steroids are administered via the inhalation route. Beclomethasone, fluticasone, and budesonide are the most commonly used inhalational drugs.
- Severe cases of asthma, which do not respond to inhaled steroids, may require administration of oral corticosteroids, such as prednisolone or methylprednisolone. This will require tapering prior to switching to inhaled steroids. Oral steroids are also used in status asthmaticus.

Leukotriene antagonists:

- As the name suggests, these drugs exert an anti-inflammatory effect by blocking the leukotriene pathway. The mechanism of action varies. Drugs like montelukast and zafirlukast act by binding to the leukotriene receptor and exerting antagonist effect. Zileuton inhibits the enzyme lipoxygenase.

- Inhibition of leukotrienes suppresses inflammation and also promotes bronchodilation.

- These drugs are absorbed from the oral route and are highly bound to plasma proteins. They are metabolized in the liver. Zileuton is excreted in the urine and the other two undergo biliary excretion. The plasma half-life is short for montelukast (3-4 hours) and longer for zafirlukast (8-12 hours).

- They can be used as alternatives to glucocorticoids in mild-to-moderate asthma. In severe asthma, they can be added to glucocorticoids and can facilitate dose reduction.

- Adverse effects include headache, rashes, eosinophilia, and neuropathy.

Mast cell stabilizers:

- Cromolyn sodium is a drug that prevents degranulation of mast cells. This in turn prevents release of histamine, interleukins, and leukotrienes, thus exerting an anti-inflammatory effect.

- It does not have bronchodilator activity. It can be used as a long-term prophylactic agent in asthma.

Anti-IgE antibody:

- Omalizumab is an IgE antibody derived from recombinant DNA. By binding to IgE, it decreases antigen binding to mast cells and basophils, thus limiting the allergic and inflammatory response.

- It is used in moderate to severe asthma that does not respond to steroid therapy.

- Adverse effects include fever, rashes, arthralgia, and sometimes, anaphylaxis.

EXERCISES

1. Which of the following antitussives acts at the peripheral nervous system?
   a. Codeine
   b. Ethylmorphine
   c. Dextromethorphan
   d. Benzonatate

2. Which expectorant liquefies mucus by breaking disulfide bonds?
   a. Guaifenesin
   b. Ambroxol
   c. Acetylcysteine
   d. Bromhexine

3. Which of the following is usually not a component of pharyngeal demulcents?
   a. Benzocaine
   b. Codeine
   c. Peppermint oil
   d. Dextromethorphan

4. Which of the following drugs is used for acute symptomatic relief from asthma?
   a. Albuterol
   b. Salmeterol
   c. Theophylline
   d. Budesonide

5. Which of the following bronchodilators has an antiinflammatory effect?
   a. Theophylline
   b. Ipratropium bromide
   c. Albuterol
   d. Formoterol

6. What is the first choice of drug therapy for maintenance in a patient with persistent asthma?

a. Beta agonists
b. Methylxanthines
c. Corticosteroids
d. Leukotriene antagonists

7. Which of the following drugs inhibits the enzyme lipoxygenase?
    a. Zafirlukast
    b. Zileuton
    c. Montelukast
    d. Cromolyn sodium

8. What is the half-life of montelukast?
    a. 1-2 hours
    b. 3-4 hours
    c. 5-6 hours
    d. 7-8 hours

9. Which of the following drugs inhibits degranulation of mast cells?
    a. Budesonide
    b. Cromolyn sodium
    c. Montelukast
    d. Omalizumab

10. Which of the following drugs acts by decreasing antigen binding to mast cells?
    a. Budesonide
    b. Cromolyn sodium
    c. Montelukast
    d. Omalizumab

UNIT IX : GASTROINTESTINAL SYSTEM

CHAPTER 1

Drugs Used for Diseases of the GI Tract

Diseases of the gastrointestinal tract fall under four main categories – gastric ulcer disease, emesis, diarrhea, and constipation.

DRUGS USED FOR PEPTIC ULCER AND GASTRO-ESOPHAGEAL REFLUX DISEASE

Gastric or peptic ulcers are formed when the gastric mucosa is directly exposed to acidic secretions. This can occur when there is an increase in aggressive factors, including acid, pepsin, bile, and the micro-organism Helicobacter pylori; or a decrease in defensive factors, including gastric mucous, bicarbonate, and prostaglandins. Gastric acid secretion is usually stimulated by histamine, acetylcholine, and gastrin, and inhibited by prostaglandins. To address these factors, various drugs are used in the management of peptic ulcer disease.

H2 antagonists:
- These drugs block histamine type 2 receptors in the stomach, and decrease gastric acid production.
- They are indicated for gastric and duodenal ulcers, as well as gastritis.
- The four main drugs in this category are cimetidine, ranitidine, famotidine, and nizatidine.

Proton pump inhibitors:
- As the name suggests, these drugs covalently bind to the proton pump (H+/K+ ATPase system) and inactivate it. The proton pump secretes hydrogen ions into the gastric lumen, for acid secretion. Therefore, these drugs ultimately suppress gastric acid secretion.
- The various drugs used in this category include omeprazole, lansoprazole, rabeprazole, and pantoprazole.
- These drugs are effective when taken orally, however, they are usually enteric coated to avoid transformation in the gastric juice. They must preferably be

taken 30 to 60 minutes before meals. They are metabolized quickly in the liver and excreted in urine. Although the plasma t ½ is only 1-2 hours, the effect lasts for 2-3 days because of covalent binding to the enzyme.

- PPIs are the preferred drug of choice for management of ulcers, GERD, esophagitis, and hypersecretory conditions like Zollinger-Ellison syndrome.
- Adverse effects include vitamin B12 deficiency, hypomagnesemia, diarrhea, and Cl. difficile colitis. Long-term use may increase the risk of fractures. PPIs must never be given to patients taking clopidogrel, as it can increase the risk of cardiovascular events.

Prostaglandin analogues:
- Misoprostol is a synthetic analogue of PGE1.
- It stimulates gastric mucous and bicarbonate secretion, inhibits gastric acid secretion, and therefore exerts a protective effect on gastric mucosa.
- It is indicated as prophylaxis for ulcers in patients taking NSAIDS. It is contraindicated in pregnant patients as it can induce uterine contractions.
- Adverse effects include nausea and diarrhea.

Antacids:
- These are substances with high pH (bases) that work by neutralizing gastric acid. They neutralize existing acid and do not prevent secretion of new acid. Over time, excess acid may be produced to compensate for the neutral effect, leading to an acid rebound. They are mostly used to provide immediate symptomatic relief.
- Magnesium hydroxide (milk of magnesia), aluminum hydroxide, and calcium carbonate are commonly used antacids. They must ideally be taken after meals as they act immediately, and are effective for 2-3 hours.

CYTOPROTECTIVE AGENTS:

These drugs reduce inflammation, prevent injury to gastric mucosa, and promote ulcer healing.

Sucralfate
- This is an aluminum salt of sucrose. It has a local mechanism of action. It binds to normal and necrotic epithelial cells, forming a gel that acts as a physical barrier between the gastric mucosa and acidic secretion.
- It only acts at acidic pH and must not be combined with PPIs, H2 blockers, or antacids.
- It may be used for patients with peptic and duodenal ulcers. However, it does not prevent NSAID-induced ulcers.

226

Bismuth subsalicylate

- This drug also forms a barrier by binding with tissue glycoproteins. Apart from this, it has antimicrobial activity, inhibits pepsin activity, and increases mucous secretion.

Antimicrobial therapy:

- Several patients with gastritis and ulcers show infection with H.pylori. H.pylori plays an important role in pathogenesis of peptic ulcer, and its eradication improves prognosis for patients.

- Commonly used antibiotics include amoxicillin, clarithromycin, metronidazole, and tetracycline.

- Generally, H.pylori eradication uses triple therapy (Metronidazole or amoxicillin, clarithromycin, and PPI), or quadruple therapy (Metronidazole, tetracycline, PPI, and bismuth subsalicylate).

ANTIEMETIC DRUGS

Emesis, or vomiting occurs when the vomiting center, located in the medulla, is stimulated. Impulses to this center are relayed by two important areas of the brain - the chemoreceptor trigger zone (CTZ), and nucleus tractus solitarius (NTS). The CTZ and NTS communicate with the vomiting center through a variety of neurotransmitters, namely, histamine (H1 receptors), dopamine (D2 receptors), serotonin (5HT-3), neurokinin, and cholinergic (M) receptors. Antiemetic drugs, therefore, address one of these areas.

Anticholinergic drugs:

- Hyoscine and dicyclomine are usually used. They act by blocking cholinergic receptors.

- They are effective in preventing motion sickness, but do not have any effect on chemotherapy-induced emesis, if the drugs directly act on the CTZ.

H1 antihistamines:

- Promethazine, diphenhydramine ,and dimenhydrinate are useful in controlling motion sickness.

- Doxylamine is used along with pyridoxine for management of emesis during pregnancy.

- Meclizine is long-acting and is preferred for sea-sickness.

Neuroleptics (Phenothiazines):

- Prochlorperazine is the main drug used in this category. It blocks dopamine receptors in the CTZ.

- It is useful in emesis due to chemotherapeutic agents. However, it can cause extrapyramidal side effects like muscle dystonia.

Serotonin receptor blockers:

- They block 5-HT3 receptors both in the brain and periphery. These drugs have a longer duration of action and are commonly used antiemetics.
- Ondansetron and granisetron block emesis due to cisplatin therapy.
- They are also used in management of post-anesthesia nausea and vomiting.

Prokinetic drugs (Benzamides):

- Metoclopramide is a prokinetic drug that antagonizes both dopamine and 5HT-3 receptors. It also speeds gastric emptying by increasing gastric peristalsis and relaxing the pylorus and duodenum.
- It is useful in postoperative emesis and emesis due to cisplatin and other chemotherapy drugs.
- Domperidone also blocks D2 receptors, but it's extrapyramidal side effects are low as it does not effectively penetrate the blood-brain barrier.

NEUROKININ RECEPTOR ANTAGONISTS:

- Aprepitant is a new drug that blocks the neurokinin receptors and substance P. It is useful when highly emetogenic chemotherapy drugs are used.
- It may cause weakness, fatigue, and flatulence.

Corticosteroids:

- Some corticosteroids, like dexamethasone and methylprednisolone, can have an antiemetic effect against chemotherapy drugs.
- They are usually not used alone, but combined with other agents.

Benzodiazepines:

- Lorazepam and alprazolam have weak anti-emetic effects. They are more useful in treating anticipated vomiting, where they might be beneficial due to their sedative effect.

DRUGS USED TO TREAT DIARRHEA

Diarrhea is defined as the passage of three or more loose, watery stools in a 24-hour period. It can occur due to decreased absorption of electrolyte and water from the GI tract, inflammation of GI mucosa, or increased motility of the GI tract. The following categories of drugs are used to manage diarrhea:

Antimotility drugs:

- These drugs are opioid derivatives. They stimulate opioid receptors in the enteric system, which reduces propulsive movements of the intestine, increase absorption, and diminish intestinal secretions.
- Common drugs used are loperamide and diphenoxylate, which are derivatives of meperidine.
- This can cause abdominal cramps, rashes, and intestinal paresis. There is a risk of toxic megacolon in patients who have colitis.

Adsorbents:

- Drugs like aluminum oxide and methylcellulose act locally by absorbing toxins and micro-organisms, and by coating the intestinal mucosa.
- They can improve consistency of the stools and ease abdominal pain.

Agents to improve fluid and electrolyte transport:

- Bismuth subsalicylate decreases fluid secretion in the bowel. It is also useful in management of traveler's diarrhea.

DRUGS USED FOR THE MANAGEMENT OF CONSTIPATION

Drugs that are used to treat constipation are referred to as laxatives. Several classes of drugs may be used as laxatives:

Stimulant drugs:

- These drugs act by irritating the intestinal mucosa and stimulating motility.
- Diphenyl methanes such as bisacodyl and phenolphthalein act by increasing nitric oxide secretion, which acts on nerve fibers in the colon. They cause evacuation in 3 to 4 hours.
- Senna is a plant product derived from the cassia plant. It can cause evacuation in 8 to 10 hours. It is useful in opioid-induced constipation.
- Castor oil is a natural laxative. It is broken down in the small intestine to ricinoleic acid, which is a powerful irritant and stimulates bowel movements in 2-3 hours.
- Irritant laxatives can cause cramping and abdominal pain.

Bulk laxatives:

- These are hydrophilic colloids which react with water in the large intestine to form gels. This increases the bulk of stools and promotes evacuation.

- Bran, psyllium husk, and methylcellulose are examples of bulk laxatives. These compounds must be taken with plenty of water, otherwise they have the potential to cause intestinal obstruction. They may cause flatulence.

Stool softeners and lubricants:

- These are detergent like substances that react with the stools to make them softer. This eases their passage through the digestive tract.
- Docusate sodium and docusate calcium are commonly used stool softeners. They may cause nausea, cramps, and abdominal pain.
- Liquid paraffin, mineral oils, and glycerin are lubricants, which ease the passage of stools through the intestine.

Chloride channel activators:

- Drugs such as lubiprostone activate chloride channels, which increases fluid secretion into the intestinal lumen.
- It is quickly metabolized in the stomach and jejunum.
- Tolerance usually does not develop to this drug, and hence it is useful in chronic constipation.

EXERCISES

1. Which of the following drugs must not be used in patients taking PPIs to avoid cardiovascular events?
   a. Aspirin
   b. Clopidogrel
   c. Digoxin
   d. Amiodarone

2. Sucralfate is a combination of sucrose and salt of which of the following metals?
   a. Sodium
   b. Potassium
   c. Aluminum
   d. Calcium

3. Which of the following is a prostaglandin analogue?
   a. Ondansetron
   b. Misoprostol
   c. Meperidine
   d. Lubiprostone

4. Which of the following antihistamines is preferred for morning sickness?
   a. Doxylamine
   b. Promethazine
   c. Meclizine
   d. Cetirizine

5. Which of the following drugs are effective in nausea against cisplatin therapy?
   a. Diphenhydramine
   b. Ondansetron
   c. Domperidone
   d. Dexamethasone

6. Which of the following drugs is an antagonist for neurokinin?
   a. Metoclopramide
   b. Granisetron
   c. Aprepitant
   d. Lorazepam

7. Which of the following drugs is not a part of triple therapy?
   a. Amoxicillin
   b. Clarithromycin
   c. Omeprazole
   d. Bismuth subsalicylate

8. Which of the following drugs is used in the management of traveler's diarrhea?
   a. Loperamide
   b. Bismuth subsalicylate
   c. Meperidine
   d. Aluminum oxide

9. Which of the following drugs stimulates intestinal motility?
   a. Bisacodyl
   b. Psyllium
   c. Docusate
   d. Lubiprostone

10. Which of the following drugs is most useful for chronic constipation?
   a. Ondansetron
   b. Misoprostol
   c. Meperidine
   d. Lubiprostone

UNIT X : GENITOURINARY SYSTEM

Diuretics

Diuretics are drugs which increase urine output. Usually, these drugs cause a net loss of both sodium and water in urine. Based on their efficacy, they may be categorized as high ceiling, medium efficacy, and weak diuretics.

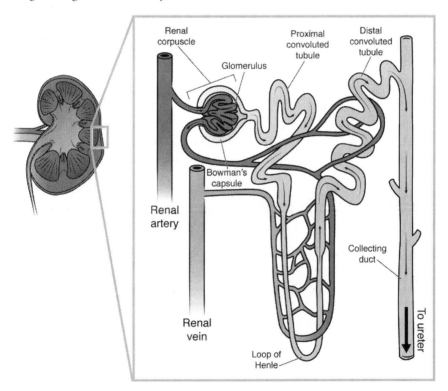

Figure 10 Nephrons are functional units within the kidney, and are the structures that produce urine in the process of removing waste and excess substances from the blood.

HIGH CEILING DIURETICS/LOOP DIURETICS:

- These drugs have maximum diuretic effect and produce large amounts of urine. Diuresis increases with increasing dose, and the drug is effective in patients with renal failure.

- **Mechanism of action**: These drugs act at the loop of Henle. They inhibit the co-transport of Na+/K+/2Cl- in this region. These ions are not reabsorbed, and are excreted along with water. They also improve renal blood flow.

- **Pharmacokinetics**: These drugs are usually taken orally, and have a bioavailability ranging from 60% for furosemide, to 100% for bumetanide. They are highly bound to plasma proteins, and are metabolized in the liver by glucuronide conjugation. The drugs are mostly excreted in urine, but small amounts may also be excreted in bile.

- **Indications**:
  o To reduce edema of hepatic, renal, or cardiac origin. It is used to manage heart failure.
  o Acute pulmonary edema
  o Cerebral edema
  o To manage hypertension in patients with renal insufficiency
  o To manage hypercalcemia and hyperkalemia

- **Adverse effects**: They have the potential to cause ototoxicity. They can cause hypokalemia, hypomagnesemia, and even acute hypovolemia. Hyperuricemia may also occur, which may lead to gout.

MEDIUM EFFICACY DIURETICS

These include thiazide and thiazide-like diuretics

Thiazide diuretics:

- Thiazide diuretics include the drugs chlorothiazide and hydrochlorothiazide. There is a separate group of drugs, called thiazide-like diuretics, which have a different chemical structure, but have the same clinical actions and adverse effect profiles. This group includes the drugs chlorthalidone, metolazone, and indapamide.

- **Mechanism of action**: These drugs act on the ascending loop of Henle and the distal convoluted tubule. They inhibit the Na+/Cl- cotransporter, and inhibit sodium reabsorption. Excretion of sodium and chloride is increased. With prolonged use, potassium ions may be exchanged for sodium, leading to potassium loss as well. However, there is reabsorption of calcium ions.

- Initially, thiazide diuretics decrease blood pressure by increasing urine output and thereby reducing blood volume. Over time, the body compensates and there is volume recovery. However, they also cause arteriolar smooth muscle relaxation and decrease in peripheral vascular resistance. Therefore, the anti-hypertensive effect is maintained.

- **Pharmacokinetics**: These drugs are well absorbed through the oral route. The onset of action starts in one hour, and can last up to 48 hours. They undergo very little hepatic transformation and are usually excreted unchanged.

- **Indications**:
  o Hypertension: Mild to moderate hypertension can be managed with thiazides alone.
  o May be added to loop diuretics to manage heart failure.
  o Diabetes insipidus: They promote excretion of hyperosmolar urine.
  o Hypercalciuria: They prevent excess excretion of calcium in urine.

- **Adverse effects**: Potassium depletion, hyponatremia, and volume depletion may occur. It can also cause hyperuricemia, hypercalcemia, and hyperglycemia.

WEAK DIURETICS

There are three categories of drugs which are weak diuretics – potassium-sparing diuretics, carbonic anhydrase inhibitors, and osmotic diuretics.

Potassium-sparing diuretics:

- These drugs act at the site of the collecting ducts, where they inhibit sodium reabsorption and potassium excretion. As the name suggests, they tend to retain potassium, and therefore carry the risk of hyperkalemia. Patients using these drugs must be carefully monitored for their potassium levels.

- **Mechanism of action**: Based on their mechanism of action, there are two distinct classes of potassium-sparing diuretics:
  o Aldosterone antagonists: Spironolactone and eplerenone act as antagonists to the aldosterone receptor and prevent its binding.
  o Sodium channel blockers: These drugs block sodium channels, which decreases the exchange of sodium with potassium. This causes excretion of sodium and retention of potassium. The drugs in this category are triamterene and amiloride.

- **Pharmacokinetics**: All potassium-sparing drugs are taken orally, and bind significantly to plasma proteins. They are metabolized in the liver, and metabolites are also active.

- **Adverse effects**:
  o Spironolactone can cause gynecomastia and menstrual irregularities.
  o All potassium-sparing diuretics have the potential to cause hyperkalemia.

237

- **Indications**:

  o Diuretics: They are used in conjunction with thiazide and loop diuretics.
  o Spironolactone is used in secondary hyperaldosteronism.
  o Heart failure: They prevent remodeling of the heart and decrease mortality.
  o Used in ascites and polycystic ovary syndrome
  o Used in hypertension resistant to other medications.

Carbonic anhydrase inhibitors:

- These drugs inhibit the enzyme carbonic anhydrase. Carbonic anhydrase converts water and carbon dioxide into carbonic acid, which breaks down into hydrogen and bicarbonate ions. These drugs inhibit availability of hydrogen ions in the proximal convoluted tubule, which cannot be exchanged for sodium ions. The main drug in this category is acetazolamide.

- **Pharmacokinetics**: It is well absorbed from oral routes. It is highly bound to plasma proteins and does not undergo metabolism. It is excreted unchanged in urine.

- **Adverse effects**: Metabolic acidosis can occur due to bicarbonate excretion.

- **Indications**:

  o Prophylaxis of acute mountain sickness
  o To reduce intraocular pressure in glaucoma

Osmotic diuretics:

- Mannitol is a drug that increases the osmolarity of the renal tubular fluid. This prevents further reabsorption of water. It does not affect sodium excretion, and is therefore not useful in conditions with sodium retention.

- It can only be administered intravenously. It is excreted unchanged in 1.5 hours

- **Indications**:

  o Acute renal failure due to trauma, drugs etc.
  o Increased intracranial pressure and intraocular pressure e.g. following trauma, stroke, cavernous sinus thrombosis etc.

- **Contraindications**: Anuria and acute tubular necrosis, cerebral hemorrhage, acute left ventricular or congestive cardiac failure.

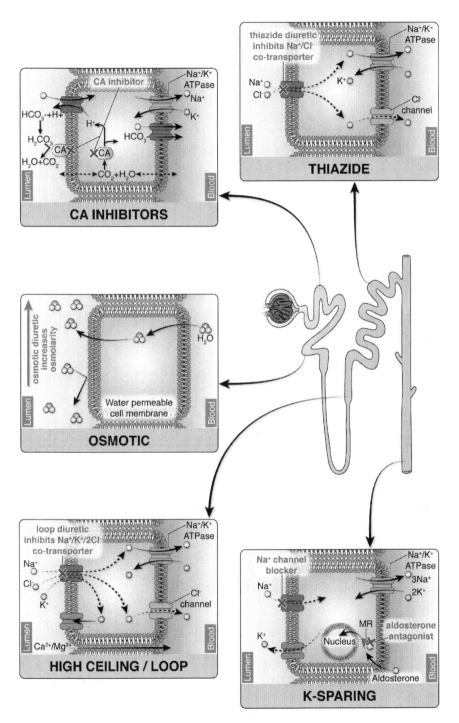

EXERCISES

1. What is the bioavailability of bumetanide?
   a. 50%
   b. 70%
   c. 90%
   d. 100%

2. Which of the following is not an adverse effect of loop diuretics?
   a. Ototoxicity
   b. Hyperkalemia
   c. Hyperuricemia
   d. Hypomagnesemia

3. Which of the following diuretics does not affect the Na+/Cl-cotransporter?
   a. Chlorothiazide
   b. Metolazone
   c. Furosemide
   d. Chlorthalidone

4. How long does the effect of thiazide diuretics last?
   a. 12 hours
   b. 24 hours
   c. 48 hours
   d. 72 hours

5. Which of the following drugs is an antagonist to aldosterone?
   a. Chlorthalidone
   b. Spironolactone
   c. Triamterene
   d. Amiloride

6. Which of the following drugs can cause metabolic acidosis?
   a. Furosemide
   b. Acetazolamide
   c. Spironolactone
   d. Amiloride

7. Which of the following drugs does not affect sodium excretion?
   a. Mannitol
   b. Spironolactone
   c. Triamterene
   d. Amiloride

8. In which of the following conditions is mannitol contraindicated?
   a. Stroke
   b. Drug induced renal failure
   c. Congestive cardiac failure
   d. Cavernous sinus thrombosis

9. Which of the following drugs is indicated for acute mountain sickness?
   a. Chlorothiazide
   b. Furosemide
   c. Mannitol
   d. Acetazolamide

10. Which of the following drugs is indicated for diabetes insipidus?
   a. Chlorothiazide
   b. Furosemide
   c. Mannitol
   d. Acetazolamide

UNIT XI : ANTIMICROBIALS

Antibacterial Drugs

Infections are diseases that are caused by microorganisms – bacterial, viral, protozoal, or fungal. Drugs used in antimicrobial therapy have the capacity to kill microorganisms without damaging host cells.

Antibacterial drugs, or antibiotics, are the most common form of antimicrobial therapy used. Different antibiotics are effective against a different range of microorganisms. Antibiotics may be selected empirically, based on previous knowledge of similar infections, or after sensitivity testing, in which infectious material (such as pus or sputum) is grown along with antibiotic discs, and the most effective one is chosen based on inhibition of bacterial growth. The usual antimicrobial spectrum of commonly used antibiotics is summarized in Table 1.

Based on their mechanism of action, there are several different kinds of antibiotics. These are described below.

CELL WALL INHIBITORS

These drugs act by inhibiting cell wall synthesis. This results in exposure of the underlying cell membrane. The cell membrane is not osmotically stable and cell lysis can occur due to raised osmotic pressure. All cell wall inhibitors are bactericidal drugs. Most of these drugs have a beta-lactam ring in their structure, and are hence referred to as beta-lactam antibiotics.

PENICILLINS:

In addition to inhibiting cell wall synthesis, these drugs also bind to proteins on the surface of the cell membrane, called penicillin-binding proteins (PBPs). This can alter bacterial morphology and lead to lysis. Penicillins are classified into the following categories:

- Natural penicillin: Penicillin G
- Acid-resistant penicillin: Penicillin V is not destroyed by gastric acids, unlike penicillin G.
- Extended-spectrum penicillins: Ampicillin, amoxicillin, carbenicillin, piperacillin

- Penicillinase-resistant penicillins: Staphylococcus produces the enzyme penicillinase which normally inactivates this drug. Methicillin, cloxacillin, dicloxacillin are resistant to this enzyme.

Pharmacokinetics:

- Some penicillins, such as amoxicillin, dicloxacillin, and Penicillin V are taken by oral route, while penicillin G and combination drugs, such as ampicillin-sulbactam and piperacillin/tazobactam are used only through the intravenous route. Oral drugs can affect intestinal flora, and their absorption may be delayed by food.
- They can cross the placenta, but do not penetrate bone or enter CSF. They do not undergo significant metabolism.
- Excretion occurs through urine.

Adverse effects:

- Can cause severe hypersensitivity reactions, including anaphylaxis, in 5% of all patients. Cross-allergy is common among all beta-lactam antibiotics.
- Diarrhea due to altered intestinal flora.
- In high doses, neurotoxicity can occur. Piperacillin and ticarcillin may also cause decreased blood coagulation.
- Methicillin has been linked to interstitial nephritis.

CEPHALOSPORINS:

These are structurally similar to penicillins. Based on their antimicrobial spectrum, four generations of cephalosporins have been introduced:

- First generation: Cefazolin, Cefalexin
- Second generation: Cefuroxime, Cefoxitin
- Third generation: Cefixime, Cefotaxime, Cefoperazone, Ceftriaxone
- Fourth generation: Cefepime, Cefpirome

Pharmacokinetics:

Only a few drugs like cephalexin and cefixime are administered orally, while the rest are administered intravenously. They can cross the placenta. Few drugs such as cefotaxime and ceftriaxone can penetrate CSF as well. They are usually eliminated through urine, except for ceftriaxone, which is eliminated through bile and feces.

Adverse effects:

Allergic reactions; cross-reactivity with penicillins may occur.

CARBAPENEMS:

- These are synthetic beta-lactam antibiotics. They include imipenem, meropenem, doripenem, and ertapenem.

- These drugs are administered intravenously. They have good penetration into the CSF even during inflammation. They are usually excreted through urine.
- Imipenem is metabolized in the kidney to an inactive form that may be nephrotoxic. When combined with another drug, cilastatin, this is prevented.
- Adverse effects include nausea, vomiting, and diarrhea. Higher doses may cause seizures.

MONOBACTAMS:

- Aztreonam is the only clinically useful monobactam. It is administered parenterally and is excreted through urine.
- Adverse effects include phlebitis, skin rash, and sometimes, liver dysfunction.

BETA-LACTAMASE INHIBITORS

- Certain enzymes called beta-lactamases may destroy the beta-lactam ring of these antibiotics and remove the antimicrobial effect. Specific drugs called beta-lactamase inhibitors bind to these enzymes, inactivating them. This protects the antibiotics.
- Clavulanic acid, sulbactam, and tazobactam are usually used for this purpose.

VANCOMYCIN

- This drug is effective against methicillin-resistant Staphylococcus aureus, and Clostridium difficile.
- It is usually given intravenously. It penetrates serous cavities and CSF. It is not metabolized and is excreted in urine. The plasma t1/2 is around 6 hours.
- Adverse effects include dose-related ototoxicity and nephrotoxicity, skin allergy, and hypotension.

PROTEIN SYNTHESIS INHIBITORS

Certain drugs target the bacterial ribosomes, and prevent protein synthesis. These drugs can bind to either the 30S subunit (tetracyclines, aminoglycosides), or 50S subunit of the ribosome (macrolides, chloramphenicol). These drugs are usually bacteriostatic.

TETRACYCLINES:

These drugs include tetracycline, doxycycline, and minocycline. They have a unique antibacterial spectrum that allows them to be used for the treatment of specific infections, including cholera, rocky mountain spotted fever, chlamydia, and Lyme disease.

Pharmacokinetics:

They are taken by oral or intravenous route. Simultaneous intake of antacids or dairy products may also be absorbed from oral routes. They penetrate CSF, saliva and tears, as well as calcified tissues such as bones and teeth. They can cross the placenta and enter fetal bones and teeth. Only minocycline undergoes hepatic metabolism, while the others are unchanged. Excretion occurs through urine, and for doxycycline, through feces.

Adverse effects:

- Gastric discomfort, esophagitis. Higher doses may cause hepatotoxicity.
- If taken by pregnant women or growing children, it can cause discoloration of primary or permanent tooth buds.
- Phototoxicity, vestibular dysfunction, and benign intracranial hypertension may occur.

AMINOGLYCOSIDES:

They are most effective against gram-negative bacilli and are reserved for treating serious infections such as Pseudomonas infections.

Pharmacokinetics:

All aminoglycosides are given parenterally, except neomycin, which is reserved for topical use. They poorly penetrate CSF, but can cross the placenta. They are not metabolized and are excreted unchanged in urine.

Adverse effects:

- Ototoxicity: The antibiotic accumulates in the endolymph and perilymph of the inner ear, and can lead to deafness and vertigo.
- Nephrotoxicity: Can cause acute tubular necrosis.
- Neuromuscular paralysis: The risk is higher in patients with myasthenia gravis.
- Topical application of neomycin can cause contact dermatitis.

MACROLIDES:

These include the drugs erythromycin, clarithromycin, and azithromycin.

Pharmacokinetics:

All drugs can be taken orally, erythromycin alone needs to be taken as enteric-coated preparations, as it is susceptible to gastric acid. These drugs tend to concentrate in the liver and tissues. Azithromycin concentrates into macrophages, neutrophils, and fibroblasts. However, there is poor penetration into CSF. These drugs undergo hepatic metabolism, and are excreted through urine.

Adverse effects:

- Gastric distress and cholestatic jaundice
- Transient deafness or irreversible sensorineural hearing loss can occur
- May be hepatotoxic in patients with liver dysfunction

CHLORAMPHENICOL:

This has the same antimicrobial spectrum as tetracyclines, but is reserved for life-threatening infections when these are ineffective.

Pharmacokinetics:

It is administered through the intravenous route. It can penetrate the CSF and is also secreted in breast milk. It is metabolized in the liver and excreted in urine.

Adverse effects:

- Anemias – aplastic and hemolytic anemia
- Can cause 'gray baby syndrome' when administered to neonates.

CLINDAMYCIN:

- This is structurally different from erythromycin but has the same mechanism of action.
- It is administered orally as well as intravenously. It penetrates all body fluids except CSF, but enters into bone. It is metabolized in the liver and excreted into the bile.
- Its main adverse effect is the development of potentially fatal pseudomembranous enterocolitis, due to infection with C. difficile following alteration of intestinal flora.

LINEZOLID:

- Linezolid is a synthetic drug which is primarily useful against resistant microbes, such as methicillin-resistant Staphylococcus aureus (MRSA), and penicillinase-resistant streptococci.
- It is given both orally and intravenously. Its exact metabolic pathway is unknown, but its oxidized metabolites are excreted through urine and feces.
- Adverse effects include nausea, diarrhea, headache, rash, and thrombocytopenia.

DRUGS THAT PROMOTE DNA LYSIS

These drugs enter the bacteria and inhibit two enzymes. Inhibition of DNA gyrase causes breakage of DNA strands, while inhibition of bacterial topoisomerase prevents release of new DNA. These drugs are bactericidal.

FLUOROQUINOLONES:

These include the drugs norfloxacin, ciprofloxacin, moxifloxacin, and levofloxacin. Moxifloxacin alone exhibits some activity against anaerobes.

Pharmacokinetics:

These drugs may be administered orally or intravenously. They are also available as ophthalmic preparations. They are partially bound to plasma proteins, and distribute into all tissues including bone, lungs, kidney, and prostate. They are excreted in urine.

Adverse effects:
- Nausea, vomiting, diarrhea
- Headache, dizziness, light-headedness
- Phototoxicity, arthropathy, and glucose dysregulation have also been reported.

FOLATE ANTAGONISTS

Tetrahydrofolate, a folic acid derivative, is essential for cell growth and division. Sulfonamides prevent bacterial synthesis of folate, by inhibiting the enzyme p-aminobenzoic acid. Trimethoprim prevents the conversion of dihydrofolate into tetrahydrofolate.

SULFONAMIDES:

These were the earliest used antibiotics and are often still employed owing to their low cost. Silver sulfadiazine cream is often employed to prevent burn-related sepsis.

Pharmacokinetics:

These drugs are well absorbed through oral routes. They bind to serum albumin and distribute throughout the body, including CSF. They also cross the placenta. They are metabolized in the liver and excreted in the kidney and breast milk.

Adverse effects:
- The drug metabolites can precipitate at neutral or acidic pH and cause crystalluria (stone formation) in the kidney.
- Hypersensitivity can occur in patients with sulfa allergies.
- Hemolytic anemia and aplastic anemia can occur in patients with glucose-6-phosphate dehydrogenase deficiency.

TRIMETHOPRIM:
- This has actions similar to sulfonamides. This drug is usually combined with sulfonamides to potentiate antimicrobial effects. The combined product is called cotrimoxazole.
- Both trimethoprim and cotrimoxazole can be taken orally. They are widely distributed, and penetrate CSF, placenta, and prostate fluid. They are excreted unchanged in urine.
- Trimethoprim may produce folic acid deficiency and megaloblastic anemia. Cotrimoxazole may cause nausea, vomiting, glossitis, stomatitis, and rarely, hypokalemia.

Table 1. Antimicrobial spectrum of commonly used antibacterial agents

DRUG	AEROBES			GRAM NEGATIVE BACILLI
	GRAM POSITIVE COCCI	GRAM POSITIVE BACILLI	GRAM NEGATIVE COCCI	
Penicillin G/V	Streptococci (except viridans), staphylococci	Bacillus, Corynebacterium, Listeria,	Neisseria gonorrhoeae, N. meningitidis	-
Extended spectrum penicillins	Same as above, and S.viridans			H. influenzae, E.coli, Salmonella, Shigella, H. pylori
Cephalosporins – 1ˢᵗ generation	Same as Penicillin G			Proteus, E.coli, Klebsiella
Cephalosporins – 2ⁿᵈ generation	Same as Penicillin G			Same as 1ˢᵗ gen, H. influenzae, Enterobacter
Cephalosporins – 3ʳᵈ generation	Less sensitive to S.aureus	Same as Penicillin G		Same as 2ⁿᵈ generation, plus Serratia and Pseudomonas
Cephalosporins – 4ᵗʰ generation	Same as Penicillin G, including S. aureus.			Same as 3ʳᵈ generation
Carbapenems	Streptococcus, Staphylococcus	Listeria	Neisseria	Enterobacteriaceae, Pseudomonas, H. influenzae, Klebsiella. Proteus
Monobactams	-	-	-	Enterobacteriaceae, Pseudomonas;
Vancomycin	MRSA, enterococcus	Corynebacterium	-	-
Tetracyclines	S.aureus including MRSA, Streptococci,	Bacillus anthracis	-	Brucella, Vibrio, Yersinia
Aminoglycosides	Streptococcus, Enterococcus (with beta-lactams)	-	-	Pseudomonas, Klebsiella, Enterobacter (especially multidrug resistant forms)
Macrolides	Streptococcus	Corynebacterium	Neisseria, Moraxella	H. influenzae, Bordetella, Legionella, Campylobacter
Fluoroquinolones	Strep. pneumoniae	B. anthracis	-	Enterobacter, H. influenzae, Klebsiella, Legionella, Proteus, Pseudomonas, Serratia, Shigella
Linezolid	MRSA, VRE, Streptococcus viridans and pneumoniae	Corynebacterium, Listeria	-	-
Sulfonamides/ Trimethoprim	-	Nocardia	-	Enterobacter

| DRUG | ANAEROBES | | | | OTHERS |
	GRAM POSITIVE COCCI	GRAM POSITIVE BACILLI	GRAM NEGATIVE COCCI	GRAM NEGATIVE BACILLI	
Penicillin G/V	-	Clostridium,	-	-	Treponema
Extended spectrum penicillins	-	-	-	-	-
Cephalosporins – 1st generation	-	-	-	-	-
Cephalosporins – 2nd generation	-	-	-	Bacteroides fragilis	-
Cephalosporins – 3rd generation	-	-	-	-	-
Cephalosporins – 4th generation	-	-	-	-	-
Carbapenems	Peptostrepto-coccus	Cl. difficile		B. fragilis, prevotella, fusobacterium	
Monobactams	-	-	-	-	
Vancomycin	-	Cl. difficile	-	-	-
Tetracyclines	-	Cl. perfringens, Cl. tetani	-	-	Borrelia, Leptospira, Rickettsia, Mycoplasma, Chlamydia
Aminoglycosides	-	-	-	-	-
Macrolides	-	-	-	-	Spirochetes, Mycoplasma, Chlamydia
Fluoroquinolones	-	-	-	Only moxifloxacin	Mycobacterium tuberculosis
Linezolid	-	Cl. perfringens	-	-	Mycobacterium tuberculosis
Sulfonamides/ Trimethoprim	-	-	-	-	-

EXERCISES

1. Which of the following penicillins is not administered by oral route?
   a. Penicillin G
   b. Penicillin V
   c. Amoxicillin
   d. Dicloxacillin

2. Which component of the bacterium is affected by beta-lactam antibiotics?
   a. Cell membrane
   b. Cell wall
   c. Ribosomes
   d. Mitochondria

3. Which of the following antibiotics is not bactericidal?
   a. Penicillin
   b. Ceftriaxone
   c. Doxycycline
   d. Moxifloxacin

4. Which of the following drugs can affect blood coagulation?
   a. Ampicillin
   b. Methicillin
   c. Piperacillin
   d. Penicillin

5. Which generation of drugs does cefoperazone belong to?
   a. 1st
   b. 2nd
   c. 3rd
   d. 4th

6. Which drug is combined with imipenem to prevent nephrotoxicity?
   a. Cisplatin
   b. Cilastatin
   c. Cefixime
   d. Cetirizine

7. Which subunit of the ribosome does erythromycin inhibit?
   a. 30S
   b. 40S
   c. 50S
   d. 60S

8. Which of the following drugs is likely to cause tooth discoloration?
   a. Methicillin
   b. Minocycline
   c. Gentamicin
   d. Levofloxacin

9. Which of the following drugs can cause pseudomembranous enterocolitis?
   a. Clarithromycin
   b. Clindamycin
   c. Cloxacillin
   d. Cefixime

10. Which class of drugs does trimethoprim combine to maximize antimicrobial effects?
    a. Fluoroquinolones
    b. Sulfonamides
    c. Macrolides
    d. Aminoglycosides

CHAPTER 2

Antivirals

Treatment of viral infections is more complicated than bacterial infections. While bacteria are separate cells on their own, viruses are intracellular parasites which use the host cell's metabolic machinery to survive. So, killing viruses may not be possible without causing damage to host cells. Antiviral drugs may only be effective during the incubation period. After clinical symptoms set in, usually the replication and dissemination of viruses may exceed the efficacy of the drug.

Antiviral drugs are classified based on the type of infection they are used to treat.

DRUGS AGAINST INFLUENZA

This group of drugs is effective against influenza viruses A and B, and respiratory syncytial virus.

Amantadine and Rimantadine:

- These drugs are effective against influenza A virus. They inhibit the M2 protein of the virus, which prevents viral release inside the cells.
- These drugs are well absorbed orally. Amantadine penetrates into the CNS, while rimantadine does not. Rimantadine alone is metabolized in the liver, and both drugs are excreted in urine.
- Amantadine can cause dizziness, insomnia, and ataxia. Both drugs can cause GI intolerance.

Oseltamivir and Zanamivir:

- These drugs act against both influenza A and B viruses. They inhibit the enzyme neuraminidase, which is responsible for releasing newly formed virions.
- Oseltamivir is administered orally. It is hydrolyzed to its active form in the liver, and thereafter excreted unchanged in urine. Zanamivir is administered through inhalation and is also excreted unchanged in urine.
- Oseltamivir can cause nausea and GI discomfort. Zanamivir can cause irritation of the respiratory tract. It must be avoided in patients with bronchospasm and COPD.

DRUGS AGAINST HEPATITIS
Interferons:
- These are naturally occurring glycoproteins synthesized in the body. They activate host enzymes, which inhibit translation of viral RNA, and ultimately degrade both viral DNA and RNA. Interferon α is available for clinical use.
- It cannot be used by oral route, and is usually administered intravenously or subcutaneously. It may also be given directly into the lesion. It is taken up by the liver and kidney cells and metabolized.
- Adverse effects include fever, chills, myalgia, arthralgia, and GI disturbances. Tolerance to these effects soon develops. However, long-term therapy can lead to bone marrow suppression, weight loss, and neurotoxicity.

Adefovir:
- This drug gets incorporated into viral DNA and terminates DNA chain elongation. It thus prevents replication of hepatitis B virus.
- It is phosphorylated to its active form and is usually excreted in urine.
- Discontinuation may cause exacerbation of hepatitis. Long-term use can lead to nephrotoxicity.

Entecavir:
- This drug competes with deoxyguanosine triphosphate and prevents transcription of viral RNA.
- It is taken orally and is excreted unchanged in the urine.

Telbivudine:
- This drug competes with endogenous thymidine triphosphate and gets incorporated into viral DNA. This prevents its replication.
- It is administered orally and excreted unchanged in urine.

Boceprevir and telaprevir:
- These drugs are used for management of chronic hepatitis C infection. These drugs inhibit serine protease enzymes, which stop viral replication.
- Both drugs can be taken orally, and are metabolized by the cytochrome P450 system in the liver.
- Adverse effects include anemia, dysgeusia, and rashes.

DRUGS AGAINST HERPES
Acyclovir and Ganciclovir:
- These drugs are phosphorylated by the enzyme thymidine kinase, which is secreted by herpes viruses only in virus infected cells. The active form competes

with deoxyguanosine triphosphate for viral DNA polymerase, and gets incorporated into viral DNA, resulting in strand termination.

- Acyclovir is available through oral, intravenous, and topical routes. Ganciclovir is available only through intravenous routes. Both drugs penetrate the CSF, are partially metabolized and excreted in urine.

- Adverse effects of acyclovir include nausea, vomiting, diarrhea, and headache. Topical application may cause some local irritation. Ganciclovir can cause neutropenia, and is reserved for cytomegalovirus infections.

Cidofovir:

- This is an analog of cytosine, and inhibits viral DNA synthesis.

- It is approved for treatment of cytomegalovirus retinitis in patients with AIDS.

- It is available as intravenous and intravitreal injections. It can also be applied topically. It can cause nephrotoxicity, neutropenia, and metabolic acidosis.

Foscarnet:

- This inhibits viral DNA and RNA polymerases. It is used for cytomegalovirus, and herpes simplex that does not respond to acyclovir.

- It is available only through intravenous route and is excreted unchanged in urine.

- It can cause nausea, fever, anemia, and nephrotoxicity.

Trifluridine:

- It is an analog of thymidine and gets incorporated into viral DNA, which prevents its replication.

- It is highly toxic for systemic use. It is only used topically in ophthalmic preparations, for treating keratoconjunctivitis caused by herpes simplex.

ANTI-RETROVIRAL DRUGS

The HIV infection is a serious infection that renders the host susceptible to a variety of opportunistic diseases. Antiretroviral drugs do not cure the disease, but can allow the host to develop a reasonable amount of immunocompetence. The process of viral replication may be halted at five different stages, and based on this, there are five classes of antiretroviral drugs.

Table 2. Drugs used in therapy of HIV

TYPE OF ANTIRETRO-VIRAL DRUG	EXAMPLES	MECHANISM OF ACTION	PHARMA-COKINETICS	ADVERSE EFFECTS
Nucleoside reverse transcriptase inhibitors	Zidovudine Didanosine Stavudine	These drugs are nucleoside an-alogs. They get phosphorylated into triphos-phates within infected cells-They get incor-porated into viral DNA and prevent chain elongation	Administered orally, and can cross the blood-brain barrier. Intra-cellular half life is 3 hours.	Lactic acidosis, hepatomegaly, bone marrow toxicity, head-ache
Non-nucleo-side reverse transcriptase inhibitors	Efavirenz Nevirapine	They bind di-rectly to reverse transcriptase and inhibit the enzyme	Administered orally, me-tabolized in the liver, and excreted in urine.	Dizziness, headache, loss of concentra-tion, hypersen-sitivity reac-tions
Protease inhib-itors	Atazanavir Darunavir Ritonavir	Inhibit HIV aspar-tyl protease. This prevents virus maturation.	Administered orally. They bind to plasma proteins, are metabolized in the liver, and excreted in urine.	Nausea, vom-iting, diarrhea, altered lipid and glucose metabolism, redistribution of fat leading to breast en-largement, and buffalo hump
Entry inhibitors	Enfuvirtide Maraviroc	These drugs bind to glycopro-teins on the host cell surface, and prevent HIV from fusing with these proteins and en-tering the cell.	Enfuvirtide is given subcuta-neously. Mar-aviroc is given orally and metabolized in the liver	At the injec-tion site, pain, erythema, and nodule formation may occur.

Integrase inhibitors	Dolutegravir Elvitegravir	They inhibit integration of viral DNA into the host cell genome.	These drugs are given orally, metabolized in the liver, and excreted in feces.	Nausea, diarrhea, elevation in creatinine levels.

NON-SPECIFIC ANTIVIRAL DRUGS

Lamivudine:

- This drug acts on two viruses – Hepatitis B and HIV. It inhibits the enzymes HBV DNA polymerase and HIV reverse transcriptase.
- It can be taken orally and is excreted unchanged in urine. Its plasma t ½ is 6-8 hours, while intracellular t1/2 can be up to 12 hours.
- It is usually well tolerated. It can cause headache, rashes, nausea, anorexia, and abdominal pain.

Tenofovir:

- This is another drug which is effective against both HBV and HIV.
- It is a nucleoside analog of adenosine monophosphate. It inhibits the reverse transcriptase enzyme.
- It may be given orally and it has a long half life. It is excreted unchanged in urine.
- Adverse effects include nausea, bloating, and increase in serum creatinine.

Ribavirin:

- This drug is effective against several DNA and RNA viruses. Its oral form is commonly used in chronic hepatitis C. Inhalational form is used for management of respiratory syncytial bronchiolitis in children.
- It inhibits formation of GTP, which is essential for viral replication. It is converted to its active form by phosphorylation. Thereafter, the drug and its metabolites are excreted in urine.
- Adverse effects include anemia and elevated bilirubin. Monitoring of respiratory function is necessary as it can sometimes cause deterioration.

EXERCISES

1. Which of the following drugs is effective against Influenza B?
   a. Amantadine
   b. Oseltamivir
   c. Acyclovir
   d. Rimantadine

2. Which form of interferon is available for clinical use?
   a. α
   b. β
   c. γ
   d. δ

3. Which of the following substrates does entecavir compete with?
   a. ATP
   b. Deoxy ATP
   c. GTP
   d. Deoxy GTP

4. Which of the following drugs is preferred for chronic hepatitis C?
   a. Acyclovir
   b. Adefovir
   c. Telaprevir
   d. Entecavir

5. Which of the following drugs is not a nucleoside reverse transcriptase inhibitor?
   a. Zidovudine
   b. Stavudine
   c. Nevirapine
   d. Didanosine

6. Which of the following drugs causes redistribution of body fat?
   a. Stavudine
   b. Ritonavir
   c. Maraviroc
   d. Elvitegravir

7. Which of the following drugs prevents entry of HIV into cells?
   a. Stavudine
   b. Ritonavir
   c. Maraviroc
   d. Elvitegravir

8. Lamivudine is effective against HIV and which other virus?
   a. Herpes simplex
   b. Hepatitis A
   c. Hepatitis B
   d. Cytomegalovirus

9. Which drug is used to manage respiratory syncytial bronchiolitis?
   a. Lamivudine
   b. Zidovudine
   c. Ribavirin
   d. Ritonavir

10. Which of the following drugs must not be used systemically?
    a. Foscarnet
    b. Trifluridine
    c. Ritonavir
    d. Stavudine

CHAPTER 3

Antifungal Drugs

Mycoses are infectious diseases caused by fungi. These infectious diseases are of two kinds – superficial conditions that mostly affect the skin, and systemic infections that can affect the internal organs. Accordingly, antifungal drugs may be administered systemically, or topically.

DRUGS FOR SYSTEMIC MYCOSES

Amphotericin B:

- This is the drug of choice for serious mycotic infections. It binds to a compound called ergosterol on the cell membrane of sensitive fungal cells, and creates pores in the membrane. This disrupts electrolyte balance and causes cell death.
- It is administered intravenously. It is a lipophilic drug and is therefore complexed with sodium deoxycholate. It binds to plasma proteins and is distributed to most body fluids except CSF. It does not cross the placenta. It is excreted in urine and bile.
- It has a low therapeutic index and has several adverse effects. Fever and chills may develop a few hours after administration. It can cause nephrotoxicity, hypotension, hypokalemia, and thrombophlebitis.

Flucytosine: (5-FC)

- 5-FC is a pyrimidine analog, which enters the fungal cell after binding to a specific enzyme called permease. Within the cell, it can disrupt synthesis of nucleic acid and proteins. It is more effective when combined with amphotericin B, as that drug increases its penetration into the cell.
- It is well absorbed from oral routes. It can penetrate CSF, and some amount is metabolized to 5-fluorouracil by intestinal bacteria. It is excreted through urine.
- Adverse effects include bone marrow suppression, neutropenia, and thrombocytopenia. It can also cause nausea, vomiting, diarrhea, and enterocolitis.

Azole antifungals:

- These are of two types – imidazoles and triazoles. Only the triazoles are used for systemic mycoses. The drugs in this category are fluconazole, posaconazole, itraconazole, and voriconazole.

261

- These drugs inhibit a cytochrome P450 enzyme, C-14 α demethylase, which blocks the demethylation of lanosterol to ergosterol. Ergosterol is an important component of the cell membrane and without it, cell growth is inhibited.
- Fluconazole is taken orally or intravenously, and is excreted unchanged in urine. Itraconazole is available for oral use, and is metabolized extensively by the liver. It is excreted in urine or feces. Posaconazole is taken orally and undergoes glucuronide conjugation in the liver. Voriconazole is available for both oral and intravenous use, and is metabolized in the liver.
- Adverse effects include nausea, vomiting, diarrhea, and headache. Hypertension and hypokalemia can occur. Fluconazole and itraconazole may cause hepatotoxicity.

Echinocandins:
- This includes the drugs caspofungin and micafungin. They prevent cell wall synthesis by inhibiting the enzyme β-D-glucan.
- They are available for intravenous use. Adverse effects include fever, rash, flushing, nausea, and phlebitis.

Table 1. Indications for systemic antifungal agents.

DRUG	MYCOTIC INFECTION
Amphotericin B	Invasive candidiasis, cryptococcosis, histoplasmosis, coccidioidomycosis, paracoccidioidomycosis, blastomycosis, disseminated sporotrichosis, aspergillosis, mucormycosis
Itraconazole	Oral or vaginal candidiasis, histoplasmosis, coccidioidomycosis, blastomycosis, sporotrichosis, paracoccidioidomycosis, aspergillosis, chromomycosis
Fluconazole	Candidiasis, cryptococcosis, histoplasmosis, coccidioidomycosis, paracoccidioidomycosis, blastomycosis
Posaconazole	Invasive candidiasis, aspergillosis, chromomycosis
Voriconazole	Invasive candidiasis, aspergillosis
Clotrimazole	Candidiasis
5-Flucytosine	Cryptococcosis
Caspofungin	Invasive candidiasis, aspergillosis

DRUGS FOR CUTANEOUS MYCOTIC INFECTIONS

Terbinafine:

- This drug inhibits the enzyme squalene epoxidase, which inhibits ergosterol synthesis. It is useful for fungal nail infections, tinea capitis, tinea pedis, tinea corporis, and tinea cruris.

- It is available for oral use. It binds to plasma proteins and gets deposited in the skin, adipose tissue, and nails. It is metabolized in the liver and excreted through urine. It is also available for topical use.

Griseofulvin:

- It inhibits mitosis by disrupting the fungal mitotic spindle. It is effective against onychomycosis, and dermatophytosis of the scalp and hair.

- From the oral route, it is absorbed and stored in the skin, nails, hair, and adipose tissue.

- It must not be given to pregnant patients and patients with porphyria.

Nystatin:

- The structure and mechanism of action are similar to amphotericin B, but the drug is reserved for topical use.

- It is effective in all forms of superficial candidiasis – oropharyngeal, vulvovaginal, and cutaneous forms. Topical application may lead to skin irritation.

Imidazoles:

- These are azole derivatives which are reserved for topical use. They include the drugs ketoconazole, miconazole, and clotrimazole.

- They are used in tinea corporis, cruris and pedis, and oropharyngeal and vulvovaginal candidiasis.

- They may produce irritation, edema and contact dermatitis.

Ciclopirox:

- This drug disrupts the transport of essential elements into the fungal cell. This in turn prevents synthesis of DNA, RNA, and proteins.

- It is effective against several fungal infections including candidiasis, tinea versicolor, tinea corporis, tinea cruris, tinea pedis, and seborrheic dermatitis.

Tolnaftate:

- It stunts fungal growth by distorting fungal hyphae. It is effective against tinea corporis, tinea pedis, and tinea cruris.

EXERCISES

1. Which of the following drugs is the drug of choice for serious mycotic infections?
   a. Itraconazole
   b. Amphotericin B
   c. Caspofungin
   d. 5-fluorocytosine

2. Which of the following azoles is not a triazole?
   a. Fluconazole
   b. Itraconazole
   c. Miconazole
   d. Posaconazole

3. Which of the following drugs inhibits the enzyme β-D-glucan?
   a. Itraconazole
   b. Amphotericin B
   c. Caspofungin
   d. 5-fluorocytosine

4. Which of the following drugs can cause both bone marrow suppression and enterocolitis?
   a. Itraconazole
   b. Amphotericin B
   c. Caspofungin
   d. 5-fluorocytosine

5. Which of the following drugs undergoes glucuronide conjugation in the liver?
   a. Fluconazole
   b. Posaconazole
   c. Itraconazole
   d. Voriconazole

6. Which of the following drugs is a squalene epoxidase inhibitor?
   a. Terbinafin
   b. Griseofulvin
   c. Nystatin
   d. Ciclopirox

7. Which of the following drugs is a topical drug similar to Amphotericin B?
   a. Terbinafin
   b. Griseofulvin
   c. Nystatin
   d. Ciclopirox

8. Which of the following drugs is effective against tinea versicolor?
   a. Terbinafin
   b. Griseofulvin
   c. Nystatin
   d. Ciclopirox

9. Which of the following drugs disrupts the fungal mitotic spindle?
   a. Terbinafin
   b. Griseofulvin
   c. Nystatin
   d. Ciclopirox

10. Which of the following drugs distorts fungal hyphae?
   a. Griseofulvin
   b. Tolnaftate
   c. Nystatin
   d. Ketoconazole

CHAPTER 4

Antiprotozoal and Antihelmintic Drugs

Protozoal and helminthic diseases mostly occur in tropical and developing countries. Most of these are associated with improper hygiene practices. This chapter discusses the drugs used in management of these diseases.

ANTI-AMOEBIC DRUGS

These drugs are effective against Entamoeba histolytica, which infects the intestinal tract and can cause dysentery.

Metronidazole:

This was primarily developed as an anti-amebic drug, but its versatile antimicrobial spectrum has led to its use in several other infections.

Mechanism of action:

Metronidazole enters microbial cells by diffusion. Anaerobic microbes possess redox proteins, which react with the nitro group on the drug to form nitro radicals. The nitro radical is cytotoxic, and destroys proteins and DNA.

Pharmacokinetics:

It is well absorbed orally. The drug distributes to all body tissues and fluids including vaginal and seminal fluids, saliva, and CSF. It is metabolized in the liver through oxidation and glucuronide conjugation. It is excreted in urine. Plasma t ½ is about 8 hours.

Adverse effects:

- Metallic taste, nausea, vomiting, abdominal cramps
- Sometimes neurotoxicity can occur.

Indications:

- Amebiasis – both intestinal and extraintestinal
- Giardiasis

267

- Trichomonas vaginitis
- Anaerobic bacterial infections, including acute necrotizing ulcerative gingivitis and dental infections
- H. pylori eradication treatment
- Pseudomembranous enterocolitis caused by C. difficile.

Tinidazole:

- This is similar to metronidazole in terms of mechanism of action and indications.
- It has a longer half life of 12 hours, and lower incidence of adverse effects like metallic taste.

Dehydroemetine:

- This was previously used to treat amebiasis, but has largely been replaced by metronidazole.
- It is administered as an intramuscular injection. It acts by blocking chain elongation and inhibiting protein synthesis.
- Adverse effects include pain at the injection site, neuromuscular weakness, dizziness, cardiotoxicity, and rash.

Luminal amebicides:

- These drugs are used for the management of asymptomatic carriers.
- Iodoquinol kills the trophozoite and cyst forms of entamoeba within the intestinal lumen. It can cause rashes, diarrhea, and peripheral neuropathy.
- Paromomycin directly reduces the population of all intestinal flora. It may cause GI distress and diarrhea. Apart from amoebiasis, it may also be used for giardiasis and cryptosporidiosis.

ANTIMALARIAL DRUGS

- Malaria is a protozoal infection caused by Plasmodium falciparum and vivax. It is transmitted to humans through the female anopheles mosquito.

Primaquine:

- Primaquine is effective only against the exo-erythrocytic forms of malaria. It is not effective on microbes located within the red blood cells.
- It is administered orally and is metabolized by oxidation. The oxidized forms are active and destroy the microorganism. Small amounts are excreted in urine.
- It must not be used in patients with glucose-6-phosphate dehydrogenase deficiency, as it can lead to hemolytic anemia in these patients. It may cause abdominal discomfort.

Chloroquine:

- Chloroquine is the antimalarial drug of choice. The malarial parasite usually converts heme to hemozoin. Chloroquine prevents this conversion, and the heme destroys the parasite as well as the red blood cell.

- It is administered orally. The drug concentrates in red and white blood cells, spleen, liver, and lung. It crosses the blood-brain barrier and placenta. It is metabolized in the liver and excreted in urine.

- It can cause headache, blurred vision, and gastrointestinal upset. It can also cause discoloration of nails and skin and pruritus

Atovaquone/Proguanil:

- This combination is used for malarial strains that are resistant to chloroquine. Atovaquone inhibits the mitochondrial processes of the parasite. Proguanil is converted into cycloguanil, which inhibits dihydrofolate reductase in the parasite and blocks DNA synthesis.

- The adverse effects of this combination include nausea, anorexia, diarrhea, abdominal pain, headache, and dizziness.

Artemisinin:

- This is used to treat multidrug-resistant malaria. This drug produces free radicals that are toxic to the microorganism. The free radicals bind to malarial proteins and damage them.

- They are available through oral or rectal routes. Adverse effects include hypersensitivity reactions, nausea, and diarrhea.

Pyrimethamine:

- It inhibits the enzyme dihydrofolate reductase in the plasmodium. The drug concentrates in blood and is ingested by the mosquito when it sucks blood. It can thus prevent transmission of the disease as well.

DRUGS AGAINST TRYPANOSOMIASIS

Trypanosomiasis is characterized by two major conditions – African sleeping sickness and Chagas' disease (American sleeping sickness). The Trypanosoma parasite initially multiplies in the blood, and then invades the CNS, causing inflammation of the brain and spinal cord.

Pentamidine:

- This drug is taken up within the protozoan cell, where it interferes with synthesis of essential components, including DNA, RNA, proteins, and phospholipids.

- It is administered intramuscularly or intravenously. It concentrates in the liver, kidney, lungs, and spleen, but does not penetrate CSF. It is excreted slowly in urine, unchanged.
- It may cause renal dysfunction, altered glucose metabolism, pancreatitis, hyperkalemia, and hypotension.
- Apart from trypanosomiasis, it is also used for management of Leishmaniasis and infections by Pneumocystis jirovecii.

Melarsoprol:
- This drug penetrates the CSF and can be used for the second stage of trypanosomiasis. It is administered intravenously, has a short half-life, and is excreted in urine.
- It can cause encephalopathy. It may also produce peripheral neuropathy, hypertension, and hypersensitivity reactions.

Nifurtimox:
- This drug gets reduced and generates oxygen radicals, which are toxic to the microorganism.
- It is administered orally. It is metabolized and excreted in urine.
- Adverse effects include hypersensitivity reactions, gastrointestinal problems, and peripheral neuropathy.

DRUGS AGAINST LEISHMANIASIS

Leishmaniasis is transmitted through sandflies. It may be restricted to cutaneous or mucocutaneous forms, or may invade viscera. Amphotericin B, pentamidine, and paromomycin may be used for management.

Sodium stibogluconate:
- This drug is administered parenterally, and undergoes minimal metabolism before excretion in urine.
- It can cause pancreatitis, liver dysfunction, cardiac arrhythmias, arthralgias, and myalgias.

Miltefosine:
- This is available for oral administration. It reacts with cell membrane phospholipids, and causes apoptosis of the microorganism.
- Adverse effects include nausea and vomiting. It is teratogenic.

ANTHELMINTIC DRUGS

Helminths are 'worms' that infest the human body. These drugs kill and expel not only the worms, but their eggs and larvae. These drugs are summarized in Table 1.

Table 1. Anthelmintic drugs and their indications

DRUG CATEGORY	DRUG	MECHANISM OF ACTION	ADVERSE EFFECTS	INDICATIONS
Drugs against nematodes (roundworms)	Mebendazole	Blocks glucose uptake and inhibits microtubules in the parasite	Abdominal pain, diarrhea	Enterobiasis ascariasis, trichuriasis, ancylostomiasis, trichinosis
	Pyrantel pamoate	It inhibits cholinesterase and releases acetylcholine, leading to muscular paralysis	Nausea, vomiting, diarrhea	Enterobiasis, ascariasis, ancylostomiasis
	Ivermectin	Increases chloride influx into the parasite, leading to hyperpolarization and paralysis	Mazotti reaction – fever, headache, dizziness, somnolence, hypotension	Onchocerciasis, strongyloidiasis
	Diethylcarbamazine	Kills microfilariae	Nausea, vomiting, arthralgia, headache	Filariasis
Drugs against trematodes (flatworms)	Praziquantel	Increases permeability of the cell membrane to calcium, which leads to paralysis.	Dizziness, malaise, headache, gastrointestinal upset	Paragonimiasis, schistosomiasis, clonorchiasis, taeniasis, cysticercosis
Drugs against cestodes (tapeworms)	Niclosamide	Inhibits phosphorylation of ADP in the mitochondria	Rare – malaise, lightheadedness, pruritus.	Diphyllobothriasis
	Albendazole	Inhibits glucose uptake and microtubule synthesis	Headache, nausea, hepatotoxicity on long-term use	Echinococcosis, cysticercosis, trichinosis

EXERCISES

1. Which group of metronidazole reacts with the proteins of microorganisms?
   a. Hydroxyl
   b. Nitro
   c. Carboxyl
   d. Sulfuric

2. What is the half-life of tinidazole?
   a. 6 hours
   b. 8 hours
   c. 10 hours
   d. 12 hours

3. Which of the following drugs is not effective for extraluminal microorganisms?
   a. Metronidazole
   b. Paromomycin
   c. Tinidazole
   d. Dehydroemetine

4. Which of the following antimalarials cause discoloration of the skin and nails?
   a. Primaquine
   b. Chloroquine
   c. Proguanil
   d. Artemisinin

5. Which of the following drugs is used to treat multidrug-resistant malaria?
   a. Primaquine
   b. Chloroquine
   c. Proguanil
   d. Artemisinin

6. Which of the following drugs may be used for the second stage of trypanosomiasis?
   a. Pentamidine
   b. Melarsoprol
   c. Nifurtimox
   d. Miltefosine

7. Which of the following drugs is effective in filariasis?
   a. Niclosamide
   b. Albendazole
   c. Diethylcarbamazine
   d. Ivermectin

8. Which drug increases chloride influx into the cell?
   a. Niclosamide
   b. Albendazole
   c. Diethylcarbamazine
   d. Ivermectin

9. Which drug is used to treat diphyllobothriasis?
   a. Niclosamide
   b. Albendazole
   c. Diethylcarbamazine
   d. Ivermectin

10. Which drug inhibits microtubule synthesis in the parasite?
   a. Niclosamide
   b. Albendazole
   c. Diethylcarbamazine
   d. Ivermectin

UNIT XII : IMPORTANT MISCELLANEOUS DRUGS

Anticancer Drugs and Immunosuppressants

ANTIMETABOLITES

These drugs have a chemical structure that is similar to normal cellular compounds, which allows them to interfere with normal cellular metabolism.

Methotrexate/Pralatrexate:

- These drugs are structurally similar to folic acid, and inhibit the enzyme dihydrofolate reductase.

- They can be administered orally, intramuscularly, or intravenously. Since they do not penetrate the blood-brain barrier, intrathecal route is employed for CNS cancers. It undergoes metabolism by hydroxylation, and it is excreted via urine and feces.

- Adverse effects include nausea, vomiting, diarrhea, and stomatitis. Rash and alopecia may occur. They can also cause myelosuppression and renal dysfunction in high doses.

- They are employed in acute lymphocytic leukemia, Burkitt lymphoma in children, breast and bladder cancers, and head and neck cancer.

6-Mercaptopurine (6-MP):

- This is an analog of hypoxanthine. It penetrates cells and is converted to 6-MP ribose phosphate. This compound inhibits purine synthesis, and itself gets incorporated into RNA and DNA, rendering them non-functional. Its analog, azathioprine, acts in a similar manner.

- It is administered orally and undergoes first-pass metabolism. It does not penetrate CSF. Following metabolism in the liver, the drug and its metabolites are excreted in urine.

- Adverse effects include nausea, vomiting, diarrhea, anorexia, myelosuppression, and hepatotoxicity.

- It is used for maintaining remission in acute lymphocytic leukemia. It is also used for management of Crohn's disease.

5-Fluorouracil:

- This is a pyrimidine analog, which enters the cell and is converted into its deoxy form. The deoxy form inhibits thymidine synthesis, which in turn decreases synthesis of DNA.
- It is administered intravenously. It is distributed to the liver, lung and kidney and is metabolized in these tissues. Excretion occurs through urine.
- Adverse effects include mucositis, diarrhea, alopecia, myelosuppression, and coronary vasospasm.

Cytarabine:

- This is an analog of 2-deoxycytidine. Within the cell, it is converted into cytosine arabinoside triphosphate, which inhibits the enzyme DNA polymerase. It is also incorporated into DNA and causes chain termination.
- It is given intravenously or intrathecally. It is metabolized by oxidative deamination, and is excreted in the urine.
- Adverse effects include nausea, vomiting, diarrhea, myelosuppression, hepatotoxicity, neurotoxicity, and conjunctivitis.

ANTITUMOR ANTIBIOTICS

These are cytotoxic drugs that primarily interact with DNA and disrupt their function.

Anthracyclines:

- This category includes the drugs doxorubicin, daunorubicin, idarubicin, epirubicin, and mitoxantrone. These drugs release free radicals, which can damage DNA, oxidize nucleosides, and cause membrane lipid peroxidation.
- They are administered intravenously. They bind to plasma proteins, and do not enter the CNS. Metabolism occurs in the liver and drugs are excreted through bile. Minimal amounts may be excreted through urine, which can cause discoloration.
- They can cause cardiotoxicity and congestive cardiac failure.
- Doxorubicin is used for management of sarcomas, breast and lung carcinomas, acute lymphoblastic leukemia and lymphomas. Mitoxantrone is used for management of prostatic carcinoma. The other drugs in this category are mostly employed for leukemias.

Bleomycin:

- This is a copper-chelating agent which cleaves DNA through oxidative processes. It is administered either orally or parenterally, and is excreted unchanged in urine.
- Adverse effects include fever, chills, mucocutaneous reactions, and alopecia. Pulmonary toxicity may also occur in the form of cough, rales, and pulmonary fibrosis.
- It is used in the management of Hodgkin's lymphoma and testicular cancers.

ALKYLATING AGENTS

These agents covalently bind to nucleophilic groups on cells and alkylate DNA, destroying the cell.

Cyclophosphamide/Ifosfamide:

- These drugs are initially hydroxylated in the liver. The hydroxylated form breaks down to phosphoramide mustard and acrolein, which are cytotoxic. The metabolites are excreted in urine. Both cyclophosphamide and ifosfamide are preferentially administered orally.
- It can cause nausea, vomiting, diarrhea, alopecia, and amenorrhea. It can also lead to myelosuppression, hemorrhagic cystitis, and secondary malignancies.
- They are used in several neoplastic diseases including breast cancer, non-Hodgkin's lymphoma, and sarcomas.

Nitrosoureas:

- These drugs, carmustine and lomustine, inhibit RNA and protein synthesis. They also inhibit other enzymatic processes within the cell.
- Carmustine is given intravenously, while lomustine is given orally. These drugs distribute widely and can penetrate the CNS. They are metabolized in the liver and excreted through urine.
- Adverse effects include nausea, vomiting, and facial flushing. They can also cause myelosuppression, impotence and infertility, pulmonary toxicity, and neurotoxicity.
- These drugs are primarily used in the management of brain tumors.

Temozolomide:

- It methylates the guanine part of the DNA chain, leading to termination. It also inhibits the DNA repair enzyme, O-guanine-DNA-alkyltransferase.
- It is administered either orally or intravenously. It can enter the CNS, is metabolized in the liver, and is excreted in urine.

- Adverse effects include headache, nausea, vomiting, myelosuppression, and photosensitivity.
- It is used for CNS tumors such as glioblastomas and astrocytomas.

MICROTUBULE INHIBITORS

The microtubules, along with chromatin, make up the mitotic spindle of the cells. Inhibiting the microtubules prevents cell replication and can be cytotoxic.

Vincristine/Vinblastine:

- Also known as vinca alkaloids, these drugs bind to the protein tubulin, and prevent its polymerization to microtubules. This results in a dysfunctional spindle, which prevents chromosomal segregation and cell division.
- These drugs are given intravenously. They are metabolized in the liver through the cytochrome P450 system, and are excreted in bile and feces.
- Adverse effects include nausea, vomiting, diarrhea, alopecia, myelosuppression, and peripheral neuropathy.
- They are used for the management of acute lymphoblastic leukemia, lymphomas, and soft tissue sarcomas.

Paclitaxel/Docetaxel:

- These drugs promote the polymerization of tubulin, leading to accumulation of microtubules. However, these are non-functional, and chromosomal segregation is prevented.
- These drugs are given intravenously, and are metabolized in the liver through the cytochrome P450 system. Excretion occurs through bile.
- Alopecia, neutropenia, and leukopenia may occur. These drugs are used for management of ovarian and breast cancers.

MONOCLONAL ANTIBODIES

- Monoclonal antibodies are hybrid forms of B-lymphocytes, and they produce antibodies against specific tumor antigens. This category includes drugs like cetuximab, rituximab, and bevacizumab.
- These drugs are usually administered intravenously. They can cause fever and chills during infusion, neutropenia, cardiotoxicity, pulmonary toxicity, and mucocutaneous reactions.

PLATINUM COMPLEXES

- This class includes drugs such as cisplatin, carboplatin, and oxaliplatin. They release a chloride group within the cell, and bind to guanine in DNA. This inhibits polymerases involved in DNA replication and RNA synthesis.

278

- They are administered intravenously or intraperitoneally. It distributes to the liver, kidney, intestine, testes, and ovary, but does not penetrate CSF.
- It can cause severe vomiting, myelosuppression, ototoxicity, neurotoxicity, and hepatotoxicity.
- These are used for solid tumors, such as testicular, bladder, and ovarian carcinomas.

TOPOISOMERASE INHIBITORS

- Topoisomerases are enzymes which prevent supercoiling of DNA and reduce torsional strain. These drugs, including camptothecins (such as irinotecan and topotecan) and etoposide, inhibit this enzyme and make DNA brittle and prone to breakage.
- Myelosuppression and diarrhea can occur with camptothecins. Etoposide can also cause hypotension and alopecia.
- Irinotecan is used in treating colorectal carcinoma, while topotecan is used for metastatic ovarian cancer and small-cell lung cancer. Etoposide is used in lung and testicular cancer.

TYROSINE KINASE INHIBITORS

- This category includes drugs such as imatinib, erlotinib, and sunitinib. These drugs inhibit tyrosine kinase, which regulates signal transduction and cell division. They are available as oral formulations, and undergo metabolism in the liver.
- Adverse effects include fluid retention, and QT interval prolongation. Erlotinib can cause interstitial lung disease. Diarrhea, fatigue, hypertension, and hand-foot-mouth syndrome can also occur.
- Imatinib is used in chronic myelogenous leukemia, and GI stromal tumors. Erlotinib is used in treatment of non-small-cell lung cancer and pancreatic cancer. Sunitinib has been used in GI stromal cell and pancreatic cancers.

STEROID HORMONES AND ANTAGONISTS

- Prednisolone is used to induce remission in patients with acute lymphocytic leukemia, and lymphomas.
- Tamoxifen is used in prophylaxis and management of breast cancer.
- Fulvestrant and raloxifene, which are estrogen receptor antagonists, are employed to treat breast cancer in patients who have hormone positive tumors.
- Progestins are used for breast and endometrial neoplasms.
- Estrogens are used in the management of prostatic cancer.

- Flutamide and nilutamide are androgen antagonists used in the management of prostatic cancer.

AGENTS USED FOR IMMUNOSUPPRESSION IN TRANSPLANT PATIENTS

These drugs are generally used in patients who have undergone renal, cardiac, or hepatic transplants. Their function is to suppress immunity, to increase the chances of acceptance of the transplanted organ. Some of the more commonly used immunosuppressants are given below:

Cytokine inhibitors:

- Cytokines are signaling proteins that play an important role in immune reactions. This class of drugs inhibit cytokines, and therefore, decrease immune reactions. Important drugs in this category include cyclosporine, tacrolimus, and sirolimus.
- Cyclosporine and tacrolimus are given either orally or intravenously. They are metabolized by the cytochrome P450 system, and are excreted in bile and feces. Sirolimus is given orally, and metabolism is similar.
- Due to immune suppression, viral infections may occur, including herpes and cytomegalovirus infections. Hypertension, hyperlipidemia, and hyperkalemia may occur. Cyclosporine can cause nephrotoxicity and hepatotoxicity.

Antimetabolites:

- Azathioprine is the prodrug that first converts to 6-mercaptopurine, and then to the nucleotide thioinosinic acid.
- Mycophenolate mofetil is an inhibitor of inosine monophosphate dehydrogenase, and blocks guanosine phosphate production. It is taken orally, undergoes glucuronide conjugation, and is excreted in urine. It can cause nausea, vomiting, diarrhea, and abdominal pain.

Antibodies:

- Antibodies produced by recombinant DNA technology may be injected at the time of transplantation. They help to prolong graft survival. Antithymocyte globulins, which bind to T lymphocytes, can cause lymphopenia and impaired immune response.

Steroids:

- Prednisolone and methylprednisolone are commonly used as immunosuppressants.

EXERCISES

1. Which of the following substrates is methotrexate structurally similar to?
   a. Niacin
   b. Riboflavin
   c. Folic acid
   d. Ascorbic acid

2. Which of the following compounds has synthesis inhibited by 5-fluorouracil?
   a. Cytosine
   b. Thymidine
   c. Adenine
   d. Guanine

3. Which type of lymphoma is bleomycin indicated for?
   a. Hodgkin's
   b. Non-hodgkins
   c. Mixed
   d. None of the above

4. Which of the following is not an example of an alkylating agent?
   a. Cyclophosphamide
   b. Carmustine
   c. Doxorubicin
   d. Temozolomide

5. Which of the following is an example of microtubule inhibitor?
   a. Methotrexate
   b. Lomustine
   c. Paclitaxel
   d. Cisplatin

6. Which of the following is an adverse effect associated with all anti-cancer drugs?
   a. Nausea
   b. Alopecia
   c. Myelosuppression
   d. All of the above

7. Which of the following hormones is not used for the management of breast cancer?
   a. Raloxifene
   b. Progestins
   c. Estrogens
   d. Tamoxifen

8. What viral infections are common after immunosuppressant therapy?
   a. Herpes
   b. HIV
   c. Rotavirus
   d. Influenza

9. Which of the following proteins is suppressed by cyclosporine?
   a. Prostaglandins
   b. Cytokines
   c. Leukotrienes
   d. Histamines

10. Which of the following steroids is most commonly used as an anti-cancer drug and immunosuppressant?
    a. Dexamethasone
    b. Hydrocortisone
    c. Prednisolone
    d. Mometasone

APPENDIX

Important Drug Interactions

DRUG CATEGORY	NAME OF DRUG	CONCOMITANT DRUGS TO AVOID	EFFECT IF COMBINED
Anti-hypertensives	Clonidine	Propranolol	Hypertension
Anti-anginal and cardiac drugs	Digoxin	Quinidine	Increased digoxin levels and toxicity
Anticoagulants	Warfarin	Antibiotics – Clarithromycin, erythromycin, ciprofloxacin, metronidazole, cotrimoxazole	Warfarin effect is potentiated because they inhibit gut flora, which produce vitamin K.
		Aspirin, NSAIDS, paracetamol	Increased bleeding and INR
Antiplatelet drugs	Aspirin, Clopidogrel	Methicillin, carbenicillin	Additive platelet action, increased bleeding risk
Oral hypoglycemic drugs	Sulfonylureas	Sulfonamides	Inhibition of metabolism, hypoglycemia
Oral contraceptives		Most Antibiotics, Rifampicin, troglitazone	Decreases effectiveness of contraception
Antiepileptic	Carbamazepine, phenytoin, phenobarbitone	Cimetidine, erythromycin, clarithromycin, fluconazole.	Increases drug levels
	Carbamazepine, phenytoin, phenobarbitone	Rifampicin	Decreased drug levels

Anti-Parkinsonism	Lithium	NSAIDS, diuretics, metronidazole, tinidazole	Increased drug levels
	Bromocriptine	Pseudoephedrine	Peripheral vasoconstriction, seizures, ventricular tachycardia
Antidepressants	SSRIs	Tricyclic antidepressants	Potentiates action of tricyclic antidepressants
		MAO inhibitors	Hypertensive crisis
		Other SSRIs, SNRIs, tramadol	Serotonin syndrome, seizures
Drugs for asthma	Theophylline	Ciprofloxacin, norfloxacin, pefloxacin	Increase in theophylline levels
Diuretics	Thiazides	Sulfonamides	Can cause thrombocytopenia
Antibiotics	Penicillin, ampicillin, cephalosporins	Probenecid	Prolonged antibiotic action
	Ampicillin	Allopurinol	Can cause rashes
	Metronidazole, tinidazole, cefoperazone	Alcohol	Disulfiram-like reactions
Immunosuppressant drugs	Cisapride	Erythromycin, clarithromycin, azole antifungals, antivirals, Class I and II anti-arrhythmic agents	Metabolism is inhibited, which can lead to prolonged QT interval and arrhythmias
	6-mercaptopurine, azathioprine	Allopurinol	Increased drug levels

Pregnancy Classification of Drugs

DRUG CATEGORY	DESCRIPTION
A	Adequate and well-controlled studies have failed to demonstrate a risk to the fetus in the first trimester of pregnancy. There is no evidence of risk in later trimesters.
B	Animal reproduction studies have failed to demonstrate a risk to the fetus and there are no adequate and well-controlled studies in pregnant women.
C	Animal reproduction studies have shown an adverse effect on the fetus and there are no adequate and well-controlled studies in humans, but potential benefits may warrant use of the drug in pregnant women despite potential risks.
D	There is positive evidence of human fetal risk based on adverse reaction data from investigational or marketing experience or studies in humans, but potential benefits may warrant use of the drug in pregnant women despite potential risks.
X	Studies in animals or humans have demonstrated fetal abnormalities and/or there is positive evidence of human fetal risk based on adverse reaction data from investigational or marketing experience, and the risks involved in use of the drug in pregnant women clearly outweigh potential benefits

Source: Content and Format of Labeling for Human Prescription Drug and Biological Products; Requirements for Pregnancy and Lactation Labeling (Federal Register/Vol. 73, No. 104/Thursday, May 29, 2008)

APPENDIX III

Examples of Commonly Used Drugs Classified According to Pregnancy Categories

COMMON TYPES OF DRUGS PRESCRIBED DURING PREGNANCY					
DRUG	**A**	**B**	**C**	**D**	**X**
Antiemetics	Doxylamine, dextromethorphan	Metoclopramide, ondansetron, dimenhydrinate			
Other GI drugs	Bisacodyl	Loperamide, pantoprazole, psyllium husk, ranitidine, cimetidine			
Antibiotics		Most beta-lactam antibiotics, erythromycin, azithromycin, clindamycin, metronidazole, aztreonam, meropenem		Aminoglycosides, tetracyclines	

Antivirals, antifungal, anthelmintic drugs		Acyclovir, famciclovir, Amphotericin B, Clotrimazole, Terbinafine, Praziquantel	Fluconazole, voriconazole, hydroxychloroquine, primaquine	Ribavirin, griseofulvin
Drugs that affect endocrine system	Levothyroxine		Hydrocortisone	
Analgesics and antipyretics		Paracetamol, Indomethacin, ketamine, meperidine	Ibuprofen, most NSAIDS* (only in third trimester, else Category C)	
Anti-hypertensives		Hydrochlorothiazide, amiloride, sotalol, epoprostenol	ACE inhibitors, angiotensin receptor blockers, amiodarone	
Antiplatelets and anticoagulants		Clopidogrel, fondaparinux, apixaban, enoxaparin	Warfarin, Edoxaban	
Drugs for asthma		Ipratropium, budesonide, montelukast,		
Oral hypoglycemic drugs		Metformin		
Antiepileptic, other CNS drugs				Sodium valproate

Category C includes many of the drugs not mentioned above.

References

UNIT I - THE BASICS
CHAPTER 1 - ROUTES OF DRUG ADMINISTRATION
1. Whalen K. Lippincott illustrated reviews: pharmacology. Lippincott Williams & Wilkins; 2018 Aug 14.
2. Tripathi KD. Essentials of medical pharmacology. JP Medical Ltd; 2013 Sep 30.
3. Verma P, Thakur AS, Deshmukh K, Jha AK, Verma S. Routes of drug administration. International Journal of Pharmaceutical Studies and Research. 2010 Nov;1(1):54-9.
4. Gould T, Roberts RJ. Therapeutic problems arising from the use of the intravenous route for drug administration. The Journal of pediatrics. 1979 Sep 1;95(3):465-71.
5. Gonda I. Systemic delivery of drugs to humans via inhalation. Journal of aerosol medicine. 2006 Mar 1;19(1):47-53.

CHAPTER 2 - PHARMACOKINETICS AND PHARMACODYNAMICS
1. Rowland M, Tozer TN. Clinical pharmacokinetics: concepts and applications. Philadelphia: Lea & Febiger; 1989.
2. Dresser MJ, Leabman MK, Giacomini KM. Transporters involved in the elimination of drugs in the kidney: organic anion transporters and organic cation transporters. Journal of pharmaceutical sciences. 2001 Apr 1;90(4):397-421.
3. Kenakin TP. The classification of drugs and drug receptors in isolated tissues. Pharmacological reviews. 1984 Sep 1;36(3):165-222.
4. Rosenbaum DM, Rasmussen SG, Kobilka BK. The structure and function of G-protein-coupled receptors. Nature. 2009 May;459(7245):356-63.
5. Dean PM. Molecular foundations of drug-receptor interaction. Cambridge: Cambridge University Press; 1987 Jul.

UNIT II - CENTRAL NERVOUS SYSTEM
CHAPTER 1 - GENERAL ANESTHETICS
1. Morgan GE, Mikhail MS, Murray MJ, Larson CP. Clinical anesthesiology. New York: Lange Medical Books/McGraw-Hill; 2006 Sep 20.
2. Chu LF, Fuller A. Manual of clinical anesthesiology. Lippincott Williams & Wilkins; 2012 Feb 20.
3. Ray DC, Drummond GB. Halothane hepatitis. British Journal of Anaesthesia. 1991 Jul 1;67(1):84-99.

4. Gupta A, Stierer T, Zuckerman R, Sakima N, Parker SD, Fleisher LA. Comparison of recovery profile after ambulatory anesthesia with propofol, isoflurane, sevoflurane and desflurane: a systematic review. Anesthesia & Analgesia. 2004 Mar 1;98(3):632-41.

5. Grounds RM, Twigley AJ, Carli F, Whitwam JG, Morgan M. The haemodynamic effects of intravenous induction: Comparison of the effects of thiopentone and propofol. Anaesthesia. 1985 Aug;40(8):735-40.

CHAPTER 2 - SEDATIVE-HYPNOTIC DRUGS

1. Hollister LE, Müller-Oerlinghausen B, Rickels K, Shader RI. Clinical uses of benzodiazepines. Journal of clinical psychopharmacology. 1993 Dec.

2. Weitzel KW, Wickman JM, Augustin SG, Strom JG. Zaleplon: a pyrazolopyrimidine sedative-hypnotic agent for the treatment of insomnia. Clinical therapeutics. 2000 Nov 1;22(11):1254-67.

3. Forster A, Gardaz JP, Suter PM, Gemperle M. Respiratory depression by midazolam and diazepam. Anesthesiology. 1980 Dec;53(6):494-7.

4. Riker RR, Shehabi Y, Bokesch PM, Ceraso D, Wisemandle W, Koura F, Whitten P, Margolis BD, Byrne DW, Ely EW, Rocha MG. Dexmedetomidine vs midazolam for sedation of critically ill patients: a randomized trial. Jama. 2009 Feb 4;301(5):489-99.

5. Maxwell LG, Yaster M. The myth of conscious sedation. Archives of pediatrics & adolescent medicine. 1996 Jul 1;150(7):665-7.

CHAPTER 3 - OPIOID ANALGESICS

1. Waldhoer M, Bartlett SE, Whistler JL. Opioid receptors. Annual review of biochemistry. 2004 Jul;73(1):953-90.

2. Yaster M, Kost-Byerly S, Maxwell LG. Opioid agonists and antagonists. Pain in infants, children, and adolescents. Philadelphia: Lippincott Williams and Wilkins. 2003:181-224.

3. Smith MT, Watt JA, Cramond T. Morphine-3-glucuronide-a potent antagonist of morphine analgesia. Life sciences. 1990 Jan 1;47(6):579-85.

4. Trescot AM, Datta S, Lee M, Hansen H. Opioid pharmacology. Pain physician. 2008 Mar;11(2 Suppl):S133-53.

5. Pasternak GW. Pharmacological mechanisms of opioid analgesics. Clinical neuropharmacology. 1993 Feb;16(1):1-8.

CHAPTER 4 - ANTIDEPRESSANTS AND ANTI-MANIC DRUGS

1. Khushboo SB, Sharma B. Antidepressants: mechanism of action, toxicity and possible amelioration. J. Appl. Biotechnol. Bioeng. 2017;3:1-3.

2. Frazer A. Antidepressants. Journal of Clinical Psychiatry. 1997;58(SUPPL. 6):9-25.

3. Peet M. Induction of mania with selective serotonin re-uptake inhibitors and tricyclic antidepressants. The British Journal of Psychiatry. 1994 Apr;164(4):549-50.

4. Jefferson JW. A review of the cardiovascular effects and toxicity of tricyclic antidepressants. Psychosomatic Medicine. 1975 Mar.

5. Shaldubina A, Agam G, Belmaker RH. The mechanism of lithium action: state of the art, ten years later. Progress in neuro-psychopharmacology & biological psychiatry. 2001 May;25(4):855-66.

CHAPTER 5 - ANTIPSYCHOTIC DRUGS

1. Brisch R, Saniotis A, Wolf R, Bielau H, Bernstein H-G, Steiner J, Bogerts B, Braun K, Jankowski Z, Kumaratilake J, Henneberg M, Gos T (2014) The role of dopamine in schizophrenia from a neurobiological and evolutionary perspective: old fashioned, but still in vogue. Front Psychiatry 5:47. doi: 10.3389/fpsyt.2014.00047.
2. Miller R. Mechanisms of action of antipsychotic drugs of different classes, refractoriness to therapeutic effects of classical neuroleptics, and individual variation in sensitivity to their actions: Part I. Curr Neuropharmacol. 2009;7(4):302–314. doi:10.2174/157015909790031229
3. Lieberman JA, Stroup TS, McEvoy JP, Swartz MS, Rosenheck RA, Perkins DO, Keefe RS, Davis SM, Davis CE, Lebowitz BD, Severe J. Effectiveness of antipsychotic drugs in patients with chronic schizophrenia. New England journal of medicine. 2005 Sep 22;353(12):1209-23.
4. Gardner DM, Baldessarini RJ, Waraich P. Modern antipsychotic drugs: a critical overview. Cmaj. 2005 Jun 21;172(13):1703-11.
5. Caroff SN, Mann SC. Neuroleptic malignant syndrome. The Medical clinics of North America. 1993 Jan;77(1):185-202.

CHAPTER 6 - DRUGS USED IN NEURODEGENERATIVE DISEASES

1. Lang AE, Lozano AM. Parkinson's disease. New England Journal of Medicine. 1998 Oct 15;339(16):1130-43.
2. Calne D, Langston JW. Aetiology of Parkinson's disease. The Lancet. 1983 Dec 31;322(8365-8366):1457-9.
3. Senek M, Aquilonius SM, Askmark H, Bergquist F, Constantinescu R, Ericsson A, Lycke S, Medvedev A, Memedi M, Ohlsson F, Spira J. Levodopa/carbidopa microtablets in Parkinson's disease: a study of pharmacokinetics and blinded motor assessment. European journal of clinical pharmacology. 2017 May 1;73(5):563-71.
4. Gupta S, Jhawat V. Pathophysiology of Alzheimer Disease: Current Drug Therapy. Frontiers in Clinical Drug Research-Alzheimer Disorders. 2017 Jul 31;6:87.
5. Vargas AP, Vaz LS, Reuter A, Couto CM, Cardoso FE. Impulse control symptoms in patients with Parkinson's disease: The influence of dopaminergic agonist. Parkinsonism & Related Disorders. 2019 Nov 1;68:17-21.

CHAPTER 7 - ANTI-EPILEPTIC DRUGS

1. Rogawski MA, Löscher W. The neurobiology of antiepileptic drugs. Nature Reviews Neuroscience. 2004 Jul;5(7):553-64.
2. Dichter MA, Brodie MJ. New antiepileptic drugs. New England Journal of Medicine. 1996 Jun 13;334(24):1583-90.
3. Perucca P, Gilliam FG. Adverse effects of antiepileptic drugs. The Lancet Neurology. 2012 Sep 1;11(9):792-802.
4. Landmark CJ. Antiepileptic drugs in non-epilepsy disorders. CNS drugs. 2008 Jan 1;22(1):27-47.
5. Czapinski P, Blaszczyk B, Czuczwar SJ. Mechanisms of action of antiepileptic drugs. Current topics in medicinal chemistry. 2005 Jan 1;5(1):3-14.

UNIT III - AUTONOMIC NERVOUS SYSTEM
CHAPTER 1 - CHOLINERGIC AND ANTICHOLINERGIC DRUGS

1. McCorry LK. Physiology of the autonomic nervous system. American journal of pharmaceutical education. 2007 Aug 15;71(4).
2. Gotti C, Fornasari D, Clementi F. Human neuronal nicotinic receptors. Progress in neurobiology. 1997 Oct 1;53(2):199-237.
3. Caulfield MP. Muscarinic receptors—characterization, coupling and function. Pharmacology & therapeutics. 1993 Jan 1;58(3):319-79.
4. Pascuzzi RM. The edrophonium test. InSeminars in neurology 2003 (Vol. 23, No. 01, pp. 083-088). Copyright© 2002 by Thieme Medical Publishers, Inc., 333 Seventh Avenue, New York, NY 10001, USA. Tel.:+ 1 (212) 584-4662.
5. Ali–melkkilä T, Kanto J, Iisalo E. Pharmacokinetics and related pharmacodynamics of anticholinergic drugs. Acta Anaesthesiologica Scandinavica. 1993 Oct;37(7):633-42.

CHAPTER 2 - ADRENERGIC AND ANTI-ADRENERGIC DRUGS

1. Berthelsen S, Pettinger WA. A functional basis for classification of α-adrenergic receptors. Life sciences. 1977 Sep 1;21(5):595-606.
2. Kamibayashi T, Maze M. Clinical uses of α2-adrenergic agonists. Anesthesiology: The Journal of the American Society of Anesthesiologists. 2000 Nov 1;93(5):1345-9.
3. Sulzer D, Sonders MS, Poulsen NW, Galli A. Mechanisms of neurotransmitter release by amphetamines: a review. Progress in neurobiology. 2005 Apr 1;75(6):406-33.
4. Wiysonge CS, Bradley HA, Volmink J, Mayosi BM, Opie LH. Beta-blockers for hypertension. Cochrane database of systematic reviews. 2017(1).
5. Salpeter SR, Ormiston TM, Salpeter EE. Cardioselective beta-blockers for chronic obstructive pulmonary disease. Cochrane database of systematic reviews. 2005(4).

UNIT 4: PERIPHERAL NERVOUS SYSTEM
CHAPTER 1: LOCAL ANESTHETICS

1. Heavner JE. Local anesthetics. Current opinion in anesthesiology. 2007 Aug 1;20(4):336-42.
2. Haas DA. An update on local anesthetics in dentistry. Journal-Canadian Dental Association. 2002 Oct;68(9):546-52.
3. Becker DE, Reed KL. Local anesthetics: review of pharmacological considerations. Anesthesia progress. 2012 Jun;59(2):90-102.
4. Malamed SF. Handbook of local anesthesia. Elsevier Health Sciences; 2004 Jun 8.
5. Odedra D, Lyons G. Local anaesthetic toxicity. Current anaesthesia & critical care. 2010 Feb 1;21(1):52-4.

CHAPTER 2: SKELETAL MUSCLE RELAXANTS

1. Beebe FA, Barkin RL, Barkin S. A clinical and pharmacologic review of skeletal muscle relaxants for musculoskeletal conditions. American Journal of Therapeutics. 2005 Mar 1;12(2):151-71.
2. See S, Ginzburg R. Skeletal muscle relaxants. Pharmacotherapy: The Journal of Human Pharmacology and Drug Therapy. 2008 Feb;28(2):207-13.
3. Harden RN, Argoff C. A review of three commonly prescribed skeletal muscle relaxants. Journal of back and musculoskeletal rehabilitation. 2000 Jan 1;15(2-3):63-6.

4. Naguib M, Samarkandi A, Riad W, Alharby SW. Optimal dose of succinylcholine revisited. Anesthesiology-Philadelphia Then Hagerstown-. 2003 Nov 1;99(5):1045-9.

5. McManus MC. Neuromuscular blockers in surgery and intensive care, Part 1. American journal of health-system pharmacy. 2001 Dec 1;58(23):2287-99.

UNIT 5: DRUGS ACTING ON THE PARACRINE AND ENDOCRINE SYSTEM
CHAPTER 1: HISTAMINE AND ANTIHISTAMINES

1. Parsons ME, Ganellin CR. Histamine and its receptors. British journal of pharmacology. 2006 Jan;147(S1):S127-35.

2. Brown RE, Stevens DR, Haas HL. The physiology of brain histamine. Progress in neurobiology. 2001 Apr 1;63(6):637-72.

3. Simons FE, Simons KJ. Histamine and H1-antihistamines: celebrating a century of progress. Journal of Allergy and Clinical Immunology. 2011 Dec 1;128(6):1139-50.

4. Golightly LK, Greos LS. Second-generation antihistamines. Drugs. 2005 Feb 1;65(3):341-84.

5. Church MK, Church DS. Pharmacology of antihistamines. Indian journal of dermatology. 2013 May;58(3):219.

CHAPTER 2: PROSTAGLANDINS AND PROSTAGLANDIN INHIBITORS

1. Ricciotti E, FitzGerald GA. Prostaglandins and inflammation. Arteriosclerosis, thrombosis, and vascular biology. 2011 May;31(5):986-1000.

2. Harris SG, Padilla J, Koumas L, Ray D, Phipps RP. Prostaglandins as modulators of immunity. Trends in immunology. 2002 Mar 1;23(3):144-50.

3. Awtry EH, Loscalzo J. Aspirin. Circulation. 2000 Mar 14;101(10):1206-18.

4. Mukherjee D, Nissen SE, Topol EJ. Risk of cardiovascular events associated with selective COX-2 inhibitors. Jama. 2001 Aug 22;286(8):954-9.

5. Green GA. Understanding NSAIDs: from aspirin to COX-2. Clinical cornerstone. 2001 Jan 1;3(5):50-9.

CHAPTER 3: DRUGS ACTING ON THE HYPOTHALAMUS AND PITUITARY GLAND

1. Kazlauskaite R, Evans AT, Villabona CV, Abdu TA, Ambrosi B, Atkinson AB, Choi CH, Clayton RN, Courtney CH, Gonc EN, Maghnie M. Corticotropin tests for hypothalamic-pituitary-adrenal insufficiency: a metaanalysis. The Journal of Clinical Endocrinology & Metabolism. 2008 Nov 1;93(11):4245-53.

2. Newman CB, Melmed S, George A, Torigian D, Duhaney M, Snyder P, Young W, Klibanski A, Molitch ME, Gagel R, Sheeler L. Octreotide as primary therapy for acromegaly. The Journal of Clinical Endocrinology & Metabolism. 1998 Sep 1;83(9):3034-40.

3. Molitch ME, Elton RL, Blackwell RE, Caldwell B, CHANG RJ, Jaffe R, Joplin G, Robbins RJ, Tyson J, Thorner MO. Bromocriptine as primary therapy for prolactin-secreting macroadenomas: results of a prospective multicenter study. The Journal of Clinical Endocrinology & Metabolism. 1985 Apr 1;60(4):698-705.

4. Paradisi RO, Frank GI, Magrini OT, Capelli MA, Venturoli ST, Porcu EL, Flamigni CA. Adeno-pituitary hormones in human hypothalamic hypophysial blood. The Journal of Clinical Endocrinology & Metabolism. 1993 Aug 1;77(2):523-7.

5. Brownstein MJ, Russell JT, Gainer H. Synthesis, transport, and release of posterior pituitary hormones. Science. 1980 Jan 25;207(4429):373-8.

CHAPTER 4: THYROID HORMONES AND INHIBITORS

1. Grozinsky-Glasberg S, Fraser A, Nahshoni E, Weizman A, Leibovici L. Thyroxine-triiodothyronine combination therapy versus thyroxine monotherapy for clinical hypothyroidism: meta-analysis of randomized controlled trials. The Journal of Clinical Endocrinology & Metabolism. 2006 Jul 1;91(7):2592-9.

2. Mandel SJ, Brent GA, Larsen PR. Levothyroxine therapy in patients with thyroid disease. Annals of Internal Medicine. 1993 Sep 15;119(6):492-502.

3. Sawka AM, Thephamongkhol K, Brouwers M, Thabane L, Browman G, Gerstein HC. A systematic review and metaanalysis of the effectiveness of radioactive iodine remnant ablation for well-differentiated thyroid cancer. The Journal of Clinical Endocrinology & Metabolism. 2004 Aug 1;89(8):3668-76.

4. Cooper DS, Rivkees SA. Putting propylthiouracil in perspective. The Journal of Clinical Endocrinology & Metabolism. 2009 Jun 1;94(6):1881-2.

5. Chiha M, Samarasinghe S, Kabaker AS. Thyroid storm: an updated review. Journal of intensive care medicine. 2015 Mar;30(3):131-40.

CHAPTER 5: DRUGS USED IN CALCIUM METABOLISM

1. Peacock M. Calcium metabolism in health and disease. Clinical Journal of the American Society of Nephrology. 2010 Jan 1;5(Supplement 1):S23-30.

2. Strewler GJ. The physiology of parathyroid hormone–related protein. New England Journal of Medicine. 2000 Jan 20;342(3):177-85.

3. Austin LA, Heath III H. Calcitonin: physiology and pathophysiology. New England Journal of Medicine. 1981 Jan 29;304(5):269-78.

4. Lips P. Vitamin D physiology. Progress in biophysics and molecular biology. 2006 Sep 1;92(1):4-8.

5. Coleman RE. Bisphosphonates: clinical experience. The Oncologist. 2004 Sep 1;9(suppl_4):14-27.

CHAPTER 6: INSULIN AND ORAL HYPOGLYCEMIC DRUGS

1. Hirsch IB. Insulin analogues. New England Journal of Medicine. 2005 Jan 13;352(2):174-83.

2. Zimmerman BR. Sulfonylureas. Endocrinology and metabolism clinics of North America. 1997 Sep 1;26(3):511-22.

3. Waugh J, Keating GM, Plosker GL, Easthope S, Robinson DM. Pioglitazone. Drugs. 2006 Jan 1;66(1):85-109.

4. Hamnvik OP, McMahon GT. Balancing risk and benefit with oral hypoglycemic drugs. Mount Sinai Journal of Medicine: A Journal of Translational and Personalized Medicine: A Journal of Translational and Personalized Medicine. 2009 Jun;76(3):234-43.

5. Ferner RE. Oral hypoglycemic agents. Medical Clinics of North America. 1988 Nov 1;72(6):1323-35.

CHAPTER 7 - CORTICOSTEROIDS

1. Tsigos C, Chrousos GP. Hypothalamic–pituitary–adrenal axis, neuroendocrine factors and stress. Journal of psychosomatic research. 2002 Oct 1;53(4):865-71.
2. Wagner CA. Effect of mineralocorticoids on acid-base balance. Nephron Physiology. 2014;128(1-2):26-34.
3. Barnes PJ. Anti-inflammatory actions of glucocorticoids: molecular mechanisms. Clinical science. 1998 Jun;94(6):557-72.
4. Annane D, Bellissant E, Bollaert PE, Briegel J, Keh D, Kupfer Y. Corticosteroids for severe sepsis and septic shock: a systematic review and meta-analysis. Bmj. 2004 Aug 26;329(7464):480.
5. Poetker DM, Reh DD. A comprehensive review of the adverse effects of systemic corticosteroids. Otolaryngologic Clinics of North America. 2010 Aug 1;43(4):753-68.

CHAPTER 8 - ANDROGENS, ESTROGENS AND PROGESTINS

1. Mooradian AD, Morley JE, Korenman SG. Biological actions of androgens. Endocrine reviews. 1987 Feb 1;8(1):1-28.
2. Gruber CJ, Tschugguel W, Schneeberger C, Huber JC. Production and actions of estrogens. New England Journal of Medicine. 2002 Jan 31;346(5):340-52.
3. Feigelson HS, Henderson BE. Estrogens and breast cancer. Carcinogenesis. 1996 Nov 1;17(11):2279-84.
4. Schindler AE, Campagnoli C, Druckmann R, Huber J, Pasqualini JR, Schweppe KW, Thijssen JH. Reprint of classification and pharmacology of progestins. Maturitas. 2008 Sep 1;61(1-2):171-80.
5. Jordan VC, Morrow M. Tamoxifen, raloxifene, and the prevention of breast cancer. Endocrine Reviews. 1999 Jun 1;20(3):253-78.

UNIT VI - THE CARDIOVASCULAR SYSTEM
CHAPTER 1- DRUGS USED IN HYPERTENSION

1. Antonaccio MJ. Angiotensin converting enzyme (ACE) inhibitors. Annual review of pharmacology and toxicology. 1982 Apr;22(1):57-87.
2. Burnier M. Angiotensin II type 1 receptor blockers. Circulation. 2001 Feb 13;103(6):904-12.
3. Elliott WJ, Ram CV. Calcium channel blockers. The Journal of Clinical Hypertension. 2011 Sep;13(9):687-9.
4. Wiysonge CS, Bradley HA, Volmink J, Mayosi BM, Opie LH. Beta-blockers for hypertension. Cochrane database of systematic reviews. 2017(1).
5. Ernst ME, Moser M. Use of diuretics in patients with hypertension. New England Journal of Medicine. 2009 Nov 26;361(22):2153-64.

CHAPTER 2 - DRUGS FOR MYOCARDIAL ISCHEMIA

1. Abrams J. Pharmacology of nitroglycerin and long-acting nitrates. The American journal of cardiology. 1985 Jul 10;56(2):A12-8.
2. Shu DF, Dong BR, Lin XF, Wu TX, Liu GJ. Long-term beta blockers for stable angina: systematic review and meta-analysis. European journal of preventive cardiology. 2012 Jun;19(3):330-41.

3. Held PH, Yusuf S, Furberg CD. Calcium channel blockers in acute myocardial infarction and unstable angina: an overview. Bmj. 1989 Nov 11;299(6709):1187-92.
4. Ciapponi A, Pizarro R, Harrison J. Trimetazidine for stable angina. Cochrane Database of Systematic Reviews. 2005(4).
5. Lau J, Antman EM, Jimenez-Silva J, Kupelnick B, Mosteller F, Chalmers TC. Cumulative meta-analysis of therapeutic trials for myocardial infarction. New England Journal of Medicine. 1992 Jul 23;327(4):248-54.

CHAPTER 3 - DRUGS USED IN ARRHYTHMIAS

1. Nattel S. Antiarrhythmic drug classifications. Drugs. 1991 May 1;41(5):672-701.
2. Anderson JL, Harrison DC, Meffin PJ, Winkle RA. Antiarrhythmic drugs: Clinical pharmacology and therapeutic uses. Drugs. 1978 Apr 1;15(4):271-309.
3. Yang F, Hanon S, Lam P, Schweitzer P. Quinidine revisited. The American journal of medicine. 2009 Apr 1;122(4):317-21.
4. Roden DM. Current status of class III antiarrhythmic drug therapy. American Journal of Cardiology. 1993 Aug 26;72(6):B44-9.
5. Hondeghem LM, Katzung BG. Antiarrhythmic agents: the modulated receptor mechanism of action of sodium and calcium channel-blocking drugs. Annual review of pharmacology and toxicology. 1984 Apr;24(1):387-423.

CHAPTER 4 - DRUGS USED IN HEART FAILURE

1. Jackson G, Gibbs CR, Davies MK, Lip GY. ABC of heart failure: Pathophysiology. BMJ: British Medical Journal. 2000 Jan 15;320(7228):167.
2. Digitalis Investigation Group. The effect of digoxin on mortality and morbidity in patients with heart failure. New England Journal of Medicine. 1997 Feb 20;336(8):525-33.
3. Brophy JM, Joseph L, Rouleau JL. β-Blockers in congestive heart failure: a Bayesian meta-analysis. Annals of internal medicine. 2001 Apr 3;134(7):550-60.
4. Akhtar N, Mikulic E, Cohn JN, Chaudhry MH. Hemodynamic effect of dobutamine in patients with severe heart failure. The American journal of cardiology. 1975 Aug 1;36(2):202-5.
5. Faris RF, Flather M, Purcell H, Poole-Wilson PA, Coats AJ. Diuretics for heart failure. Cochrane Database of Systematic Reviews. 2012(2).

UNIT VII - HEMATOPOIETIC SYSTEM
CHAPTER 1 - HEMATINICS AND DRUGS AFFECTING BLOOD CLOTTING

1. Schafer AI. Antiplatelet therapy. The American journal of medicine. 1996 Aug 1;101(2):199-209.
2. Hirsh J. Low molecular weight heparin. Thrombosis and haemostasis. 1993 Jan;69(01):204-7.
3. Mekaj YH, Mekaj AY, Duci SB, Miftari EI. New oral anticoagulants: their advantages and disadvantages compared with vitamin K antagonists in the prevention and treatment of patients with thromboembolic events. Therapeutics and clinical risk management. 2015;11:967.

4. Hacke W, Kaste M, Bluhmki E, Brozman M, Dávalos A, Guidetti D, Larrue V, Lees KR, Medeghri Z, Machnig T, Schneider D. Thrombolysis with alteplase 3 to 4.5 hours after acute ischemic stroke. New England journal of medicine. 2008 Sep 25;359(13):1317-29.
5. Couturier R, Grassin-Delyle S. Tranexamic acid: more than inhibition of fibrinolysis?. Anesthesia & Analgesia. 2014 Aug 1;119(2):498-9.

UNIT VIII - RESPIRATORY SYSTEM
CHAPTER 1 - DRUGS USED IN COUGH AND BRONCHIAL ASTHMA

1. Rubin BK. Mucolytics, expectorants, and mucokinetic medications. Respiratory Care. 2007 Jul 1;52(7):859-65.
2. Schuh S, Canny G, Reisman JJ, Kerem E, Bentur L, Petric M, Levison H. Nebulized albuterol in acute bronchiolitis. The Journal of pediatrics. 1990 Oct 1;117(4):633-7.
3. Barnes PJ. Efficacy of inhaled corticosteroids in asthma. Journal of allergy and clinical immunology. 1998 Oct 1;102(4):531-8.
4. Greening AP, Ind PW, Northfield M, Shaw G. Added salmeterol versus higher-dose corticosteroid in asthma patients with symptoms on existing inhaled corticosteroid. The Lancet. 1994 Jul 23;344(8917):219-24.
5. Van Noord JA, De Munck DR, Bantje TA, Hop WC, Akveld MM, Bommer AM. Long-term treatment of chronic obstructive pulmonary disease with salmeterol and the additive effect of ipratropium. European Respiratory Journal. 2000 May 1;15(5):878-85.

UNIT IX - GASTROINTESTINAL SYSTEM
CHAPTER 1 - DRUGS USED FOR DISEASES OF THE GI TRACT

1. Sachs G, Shin JM, Howden CW. The clinical pharmacology of proton pump inhibitors. Alimentary pharmacology & therapeutics. 2006 Jun;23:2-8.
2. Tang OS, Schweer H, Seyberth HW, Lee SW, Ho PC. Pharmacokinetics of different routes of administration of misoprostol. Human reproduction. 2002 Feb 1;17(2):332-6.
3. Saad RJ, Schoenfeld P, Kim HM, Chey WD. Levofloxacin-Based Triple Therapy versus Bismuth-Based Quadruple Therapy for Persistent Helicobacter pylori Infection: A Meta-Analysis: CME. American Journal of Gastroenterology. 2006 Mar 1;101(3):488-96.
4. Gralla RJ, Osoba D, Kris MG, Kirkbride P, Hesketh PJ, Chinnery LW, Clark-Snow R, Gill DP, Groshen S, Grunberg S, Koeller JM. Recommendations for the use of antiemetics: evidence-based, clinical practice guidelines. Journal of Clinical Oncology. 1999 Sep 1;17:2971-94.
5. Baker DE. Loperamide: a pharmacological review. Reviews in gastroenterological disorders. 2007;7:S11-8.

UNIT X - GENITOURINARY SYSTEM
CHAPTER 1 - DIURETICS

1. Brater DC. Clinical pharmacology of loop diuretics. Drugs. 1991 Jun 1;41(3):14-22.
2. Sica DA, Carter B, Cushman W, Hamm L. Thiazide and loop diuretics. The journal of clinical hypertension. 2011 Sep;13(9):639-43.
3. Loriaux DL, MENARD R, TAYLOR A, PITA JC, SANTEN R. Spironolactone and endocrine dysfunction. Annals of internal Medicine. 1976 Nov 1;85(5):630-6.

4. Forwand SA, Landowne M, Follansbee JN, Hansen JE. Effect of acetazolamide on acute mountain sickness. New England Journal of Medicine. 1968 Oct 17;279(16):839-45.

5. Wakai A, Roberts IG, Schierhout G. Mannitol for acute traumatic brain injury. Cochrane database of systematic reviews. 2006(3).

UNIT XI - ANTIMICROBIAL DRUGS
CHAPTER 1 - ANTIBACTERIALS

1. KONG KF, Schneper L, Mathee K. Beta-lactam antibiotics: from antibiosis to resistance and bacteriology. Apmis. 2010 Jan;118(1):1-36.

2. Levine DP. Vancomycin: a history. Clinical Infectious Diseases. 2006 Jan 1;42(Supplement_1):S5-12.

3. Smith K, Leyden JJ. Safety of doxycycline and minocycline: a systematic review. Clinical therapeutics. 2005 Sep 1;27(9):1329-42.

4. Nightingale CH. Pharmacokinetics and pharmacodynamics of newer macrolides. The Pediatric infectious disease journal. 1997 Apr 1;16(4):438-43.

5. Begg EJ, Barclay ML. Aminoglycosides--50 years on. British journal of clinical pharmacology. 1995 Jun;39(6):597.

CHAPTER 2 - ANTIVIRALS

1. De Clercq E. Antiviral drugs in current clinical use. Journal of clinical virology. 2004 Jun 1;30(2):115-33.

2. De Clercq E. Antiviral agents active against influenza A viruses. Nature reviews Drug discovery. 2006 Dec;5(12):1015-25.

3. Whitley RJ, Gnann Jr JW. Acyclovir: a decade later. New England Journal of Medicine. 1992 Sep 10;327(11):782-9.

4. Sarrazin C, Hézode C, Zeuzem S, Pawlotsky JM. Antiviral strategies in hepatitis C virus infection. Journal of hepatology. 2012 Jan 1;56:S88-100.

5. Cohen MS, Chen YQ, McCauley M, Gamble T, Hosseinipour MC, Kumarasamy N, Hakim JG, Kumwenda J, Grinsztejn B, Pilotto JH, Godbole SV. Prevention of HIV-1 infection with early antiretroviral therapy. New England journal of medicine. 2011 Aug 11;365(6):493-505.

CHAPTER 3 - ANTIFUNGALS

1. Gallis HA, Drew RH, Pickard WW. Amphotericin B: 30 years of clinical experience. Reviews of infectious diseases. 1990 Mar 1;12(2):308-29.

2. Zonios DI, Bennett JE. Update on azole antifungals. InSeminars in respiratory and critical care medicine 2008 Apr (Vol. 29, No. 02, pp. 198-210). Published by Thieme Medical Publishers.

3. Graybill JR, Craven PC. Antifungal agents used in systemic mycoses. Drugs. 1983 Jan 1;25(1):41-62.

4. Gupta AK, Einarson TR, Summerbell RC, Shear NH. An overview of topical antifungal therapy in dermatomycoses. Drugs. 1998 May 1;55(5):645-74.

5. Baran R, Kaoukhov A. Topical antifungal drugs for the treatment of onychomycosis: an overview of current strategies for monotherapy and combination therapy. Journal of the European Academy of Dermatology and Venereology. 2005 Jan;19(1):21-9.

CHAPTER 4 - ANTIPROTOZOAL AND ANTHELMINTIC DRUGS

1. Gonzales ML, Dans LF, Sio-Aguilar J. Antiamoebic drugs for treating amoebic colitis. Cochrane Database of Systematic Reviews. 2019(1).
2. Baird JK. Effectiveness of antimalarial drugs. New England Journal of Medicine. 2005 Apr 14;352(15):1565-77.
3. Kennedy PG. Clinical features, diagnosis, and treatment of human African trypanosomiasis (sleeping sickness). The Lancet Neurology. 2013 Feb 1;12(2):186-94.
4. Tiuman TS, Santos AO, Ueda-Nakamura T, Dias Filho BP, Nakamura CV. Recent advances in leishmaniasis treatment. International Journal of Infectious Diseases. 2011 Aug 1;15(8):e525-32.
5. Holden-Dye L, Walker RJ. Anthelmintic drugs. WormBook. 2007:1.

UNIT XII - IMPORTANT MISCELLANEOUS DRUGS
CHAPTER 1 - ANTICANCER DRUGS AND IMMUNOSUPPRESSANTS

1. DeVita VT, Chu E. A history of cancer chemotherapy. Cancer research. 2008 Nov 1;68(21):8643-53.
2. Peters GJ, Van der Wilt CL, Van Moorsel CJ, Kroep JR, Bergman AM, Ackland SP. Basis for effective combination cancer chemotherapy with antimetabolites. Pharmacology & therapeutics. 2000 Aug 1;87(2-3):227-53.
3. Goding JW. Monoclonal antibodies: principles and practice. Elsevier; 1996 Feb 26.
4. Mijatovic T, Van Quaquebeke E, Delest B, Debeir O, Darro F, Kiss R. Cardiotonic steroids on the road to anti-cancer therapy. Biochimica et Biophysica Acta (BBA)-Reviews on Cancer. 2007 Sep 1;1776(1):32-57.
5. McAlister VC, Gao Z, Peltekian K, Domingues J, Mahalati K, MacDonald AS. Sirolimus-tacrolimus combination immunosuppression. The Lancet. 2000 Jan 29;355(9201):376-7.

Answers to Exercises

UNIT 1

Chapter 1
1. C
2. C
3. A
4. B
5. D
6. B
7. C
8. B
9. A
10. B

Chapter 2
1. B
2. C
3. C
4. D
5. D
6. A
7. C
8. B
9. D
10. B

UNIT 2

Chapter 1
1. B
2. C
3. A
4. D
5. B
6. A
7. B
8. A
9. D
10. C

Chapter 2
1. D
2. C
3. A
4. B
5. C
6. C
7. A
8. B
9. B
10. C

Chapter 3
1. C
2. C
3. C
4. C
5. D
6. B
7. B
8. B
9. C
10. B

Chapter 4
1. D
2. B
3. A
4. D
5. C
6. C
7. B
8. D
9. B
10. C

Chapter 5
1. B
2. B
3. A
4. C
5. B
6. D
7. D
8. B
9. A
10. A

Chapter 6
1. C
2. A
3. D
4. B
5. B
6. D
7. C
8. D
9. B
10. D

Chapter 7
1. A
2. A
3. A
4. B
5. D
6. C
7. A
8. A
9. A
10. B

UNIT III

Chapter 1
1. A
2. A
3. C
4. B
5. B
6. C
7. A
8. B
9. C
10. A

Chapter 2
1. B
2. B
3. C
4. B
5. D
6. B
7. C
8. B
9. B
10. A

UNIT 4

Chapter 1
1. C
2. A
3. C
4. A
5. A
6. B
7. D
8. A
9. D
10. C

Chapter 2
1. C
2. B
3. B
4. C
5. B
6. B
7. C
8. C
9. D
10. C

UNIT 5

Chapter 1
1. C
2. B
3. C
4. D
5. B
6. A
7. B
8. A
9. C
10. D

Chapter 2
1. C
2. B
3. C
4. D
5. B
6. C
7. A
8. B
9. C
10. C

Chapter 3
1. B
2. A
3. B
4. B
5. B
6. D
7. C
8. D
9. C
10. B

Chapter 4
1. B
2. C
3. B
4. C
5. C
6. B
7. D
8. D
9. A
10. C

Chapter 5
1. D
2. B
3. D
4. A
5. A
6. B
7. C
8. D
9. C
10. B

Chapter 6
1. A
2. C
3. B
4. D
5. A
6. B
7. D
8. B
9. B
10. C

Chapter 7
1. D
2. A
3. C
4. B
5. A
6. D
7. B
8. B
9. C
10. C

Chapter 8
1. B
2. C
3. A
4. D
5. B
6. C
7. B
8. D
9. C
10. A

UNIT 6

Chapter 1
1. B
2. C
3. C
4. D
5. C
6. C
7. B
8. A
9. C
10. A

UNIT 7

Chapter 1
1. C
2. D
3. C
4. B
5. C
6. B
7. D
8. D
9. B
10. C

Chapter 2
1. A
2. D
3. A
4. B
5. C
6. B
7. C
8. C
9. C
10. B

Chapter 3
1. B
2. A
3. C
4. D
5. C
6. C
7. B
8. C
9. B
10. D

Chapter 4
1. C
2. B
3. B
4. D
5. B
6. B
7. B
8. A
9. D
10. C

UNIT 8

Chapter 1
1. D
2. C
3. B
4. A
5. A
6. C
7. B
8. B
9. B
10. D

UNIT 9

Chapter 1
1. B
2. C
3. B
4. A
5. B
6. C
7. D
8. B
9. A
10. D

UNIT 10

Chapter 1
1. D
2. B
3. C
4. C
5. B
6. B
7. A
8. C
9. D
10. A

UNIT 11

Chapter 1
1. A
2. B
3. C
4. C
5. C
6. B
7. C
8. B
9. B
10. B

Chapter 2
1. B
2. A
3. D
4. C
5. C
6. B
7. C
8. C
9. C
10. B

Chapter 3
1. B
2. C
3. C
4. D
5. B
6. A
7. C
8. D
9. B
10. B

Chapter 4
1. B
2. D
3. B
4. B
5. D
6. B
7. C
8. D
9. A
10. B

UNIT 12

Chapter 1
1. C
2. B
3. A
4. C
5. C
6. D
7. C
8. A
9. B
10. C

INDEX

Tiotropium, 84
Tirofiban, 209
Tizanidine, 113
Tolbutamide, 153
Tolcapone, 63
Tolnaftate, 263
Topical, 3, 4, 5, 6
Topiramate, 68, 71
Topoisomerase inhibitors, 279
Topotecan, 279
Toremifene, 170
Tramadol, 286
Tranexamic acid, 212
Transdermal, 4, 6, 8
Travoprost, 126
Trazodone, 51
Treprostinil, 126
Triamcinolone, 161
Triamterene, 176
Triazolam, 34
Triazoles, 261, 262
Trifluridine, 255
Trihexyphenidyl, 84
Trimetazidine, 185, 188
Trimethoprim, 248, 249
Tropicamide, 84
Tyrosine kinase inhibitors, 279

U

Urokinase, 189, 211

V

Vancomycin, 245, 249, 250
Vasopressin, 136
Vecuronium, 85, 111

Verapamil, 179, 185, 194, 197
Vigabatrin, 68
Vinblastine, 278
Vincristine, 278
Vitamin D, (see cholecalciferol), 146
Vitamin K, 212
Voglibose, 155
Voriconazole, 261, 262

W

Warfarin, 211

Y

Yohimbine, 96

Z

Zafirlukast, 220
Zaleplon, 37
Zanamivir, 253
Zidovudine, 256
Zileuton, 220
Ziprasidone, 56, 57
Zoledronate, 148
Zolpidem, 37
Zopiclone, 37

JOIN OUR COMMUNITY

Medical Creations® is an educational company focused on providing study tools for Healthcare students.

You can find all of our products at this link:

www.medicalcreations.net

If you have any questions or concerns please contact us:

hello@medicalcreations.net

We want to be as close as possible to our customers, that's why we are active on all the main Social Media platforms.

You can find us here:

Facebook	www.facebook.com/medicalcreations
Instagram	www.instagram.com/medicalcreationsofficial
Pinterest	www.pinterest.com/medicalcreations

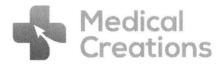

CHECK OUT OUR OTHER BOOKS

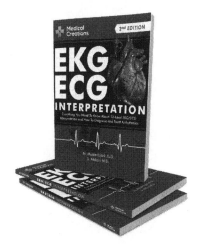

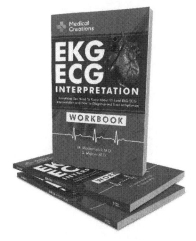

EKG/ECG Interpretation:
Everything you Need to Know
about the 12 - Lead ECG/EKG
Interpretation and How to
Diagnose and Treat Arrhythmias
(2nd Edition)

EKG/ECG Interpretation:
Everything you Need to Know
about the 12 - Lead ECG/EKG
Interpretation and How to
Diagnose and Treat Arrhythmias:
Workbook

Scan the QR Code

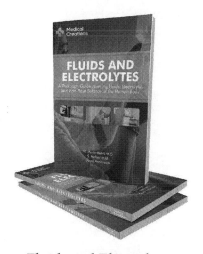

Fluids and Electrolytes:
A Torough Guide covering
Fluids, Electrolytes and Acid-Base
Balance of the Human Body

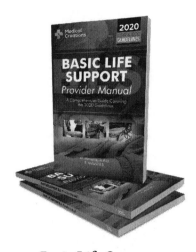

Basic Life Support:
Provider Manual - A
Comprehensive Guide Covering
the Latest Guidelines

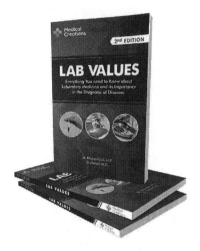

Lab Values:
Everything You Need to Know
about Laboratory Medicine and
its Importance in the Diagnosis
of Diseases

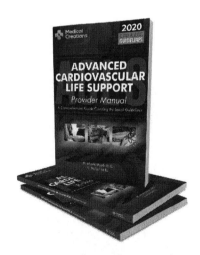

**Advanced Cardiovascular
Life Support:**
Provider Manual - A
Comprehensive Guide Covering
the Latest Guidelines

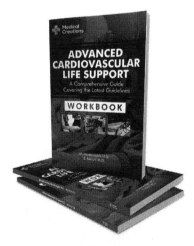

**Advanced Cardiovascular
Life Support:**
Provider Manual - A
Comprehensive Guide Covering
the Latest Guidelines: Workbook

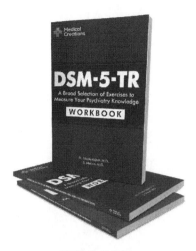

DSM-5-TR:
A Broad Selection of Exercises
to Measure Your Psychiatry
Knowledge: Workbook

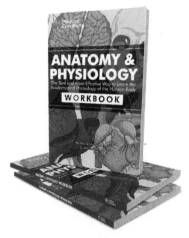

Anatomy & Physiology:
The Best and Most Effective Way to
Learn the Anatomy and Physiology
of the Human Body: Workbook

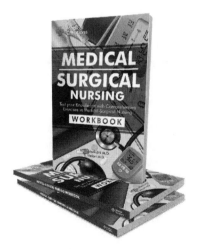

Medical Surgical Nursing:
Test your Knowledge with
Comprehensive Exercises in
Medical-Surgical Nursing:
Workbook

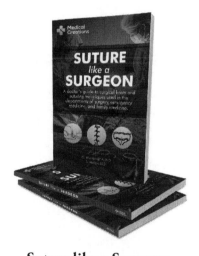

Suture like a Surgeon:
A Doctor's Guide to Surgical Knots
and Suturing Techniques used
in the Departments of Surgery,
Emergency Medicine, and Family
Medicine

Medical Creations Suture Practice Kit with Suturing Video Series
by Board-Certified Surgeon and Ebook Training Guide

SUTURE LIKE A SURGEON PRACTICE KIT

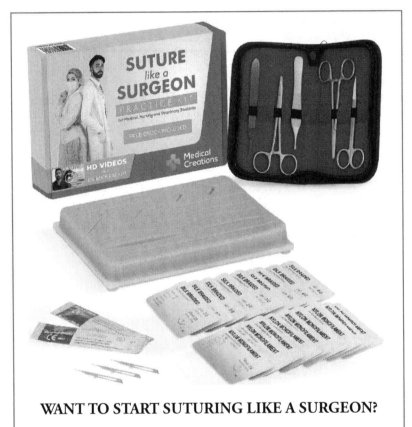

WANT TO START SUTURING LIKE A SURGEON?

Our Suture Practice Kit contains all of the tools
you need to start practicing.

Scan the QR Code

Made in the USA
Middletown, DE
05 October 2024

62057088R00181